AF564869

# Essentials of Veterinary Diagnostic Imaging

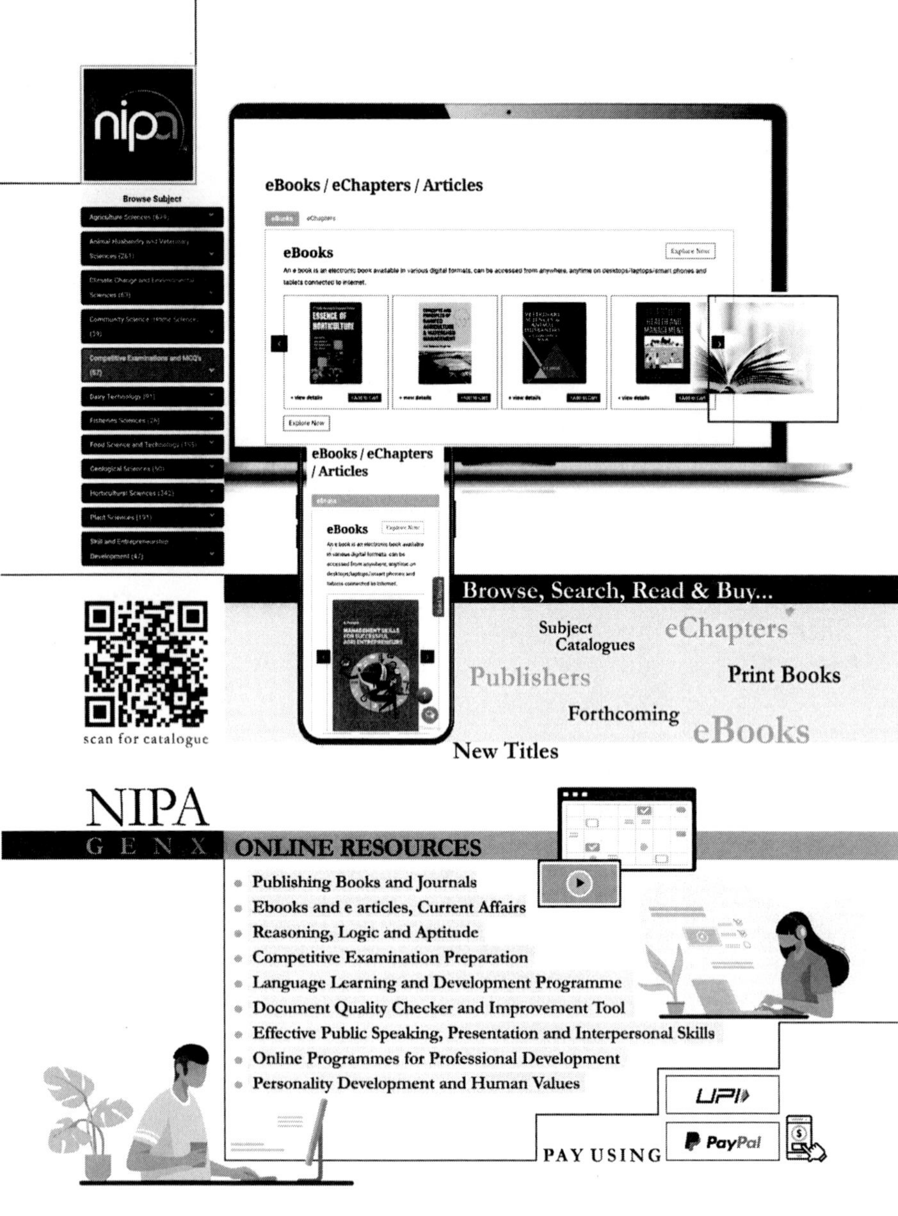

nipa
Browse Subject
eBooks / eChapters / Articles
eBooks
Explore Now
eBooks / eChapters / Articles
scan for catalogue
Browse, Search, Read & Buy...
Subject Catalogues
eChapters
Publishers
Print Books
Forthcoming
eBooks
New Titles
NIPA
GENX
ONLINE RESOURCES
Publishing Books and Journals
Ebooks and e articles, Current Affairs
Reasoning, Logic and Aptitude
Competitive Examination Preparation
Language Learning and Development Programme
Document Quality Checker and Improvement Tool
Effective Public Speaking, Presentation and Interpersonal Skills
Online Programmes for Professional Development
Personality Development and Human Values
UPI
PAY USING
PayPal

# Essentials of Veterinary Diagnostic Imaging

**( A book for both undergraduate and postgraduate level )**

**Author and Editor :**

**Dr. Md. Moin Ansari**

B.V.Sc &A.H., M.V.Sc., Ph.D., NET (ICAR), DMLT, Cert.AW, LMIVA,

Asstt. Professor -cum- Scientist (Senior Scale)

Division of Veterinary Surgery and Radiology

Faculty of Veterinary Sciences and Animal Husbandry

Sher-e-Kashmir University of Agricultural Sciences and Technology of Kashmir

Shuhama, Alustaing, Srinagar-190006, J&K

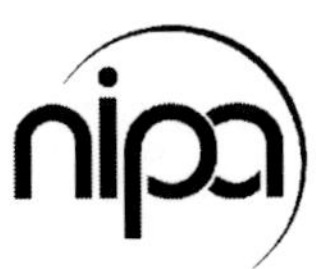


**NEW INDIA PUBLISHING AGENCY**

New Delhi – 110 034

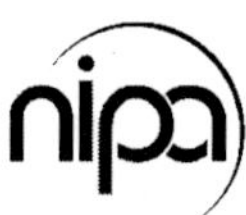

**NEW INDIA PUBLISHING AGENCY**
101, Vikas Surya Plaza, CU Block, LSC Market
Pitam Pura, New Delhi 110 034, India
Phone: + 91 (11)27 34 17 17 Fax: + 91(11) 27 34 16 16
Email: info@nipabooks.com
Web: www.nipabooks.com

Feedback at feedbacks@nipabooks.com



**ISBN : 978-93-83305-14-8**



Composed, Designed and Printed at Jai Bharat Printing Press, Delhi

***Dedicated to my first teachers…………***

***- Father and Mother***

# Preface

*"The soul never thinks without an image"*

**-Aristotle**

Radiology and ultrasound are the primary diagnostic imaging technique available to the veterinarian. The responsibility to provide useful diagnostic images usually falls on the shoulders of the veterinary radiologist/ radiographer.

The book in the concise form is a first publication on "diagnostic imaging"comprises of approximately 250 pages and runs in twenty four chapters prepared following the syllabus framed by Veterinary Council of India (VCI) will assist veterinary students in their understanding the radiology and other diagnostic imaging technology in veterinary discipline. It can act as an excellent complement to the students both at undergraduate and postgraduate level, interns, veterinarian who are called upon to diagnose an unfamiliar species.

Present book is aimed to provide a exercises: review questions, contains more than two hundred solved objective types questions, help reinforce key information for various entrance tests viz: Pre- P.G, ICAR-JRF, ICAR-SRF, NET, ARS, Pre-IAS, State PSC, State civil services examination and interviews.

At the end, available glossary literature on imaging related terms has been incorporated for the benefit of ready and quick revision. The subject matter in the book is so graded that undergraduate and post-graduate students, veterinary surgeons working in the field, teachers and as well as research scholar in veterinary surgery and those interested in the welfare of the farmers could benefit from the book.

Readers may find it helpful to refer back to those chapters if they wish to develop deeper into subject matter or reference not included in this Essentials book. At the end of the book detailed references are included for ready reference.

I wish to acknowledge the authors and publishers of different reference books consulted for the preparation of the book. Help and whole hearted support extended by the learned colleagues/ faculty members to bring out the publication are duly acknowledged.

I would appreciate to receive any suggestion and constructive criticism about the publication and our efforts would be to further improve more subject and latest information in the next edition. Hope our efforts would help to propagate the diagnostic imaging technique to the clinicians in alleviate the suffering of the animals.

At last again, I remember the almighty who gave me patience and strength to overcome the difficulties, which crossed my way in accomplishment of this endeavor.

Date: Aug. 2013 **(Md. Moin Ansari)**

# Contents

*Dedication* ........ *v*
*Preface* ........ *vii*
1. Introduction to Radiology and Historical Perspective ........ 1
2. Applications of Radiography ........ 9
3. Principles of Radiographic Positioning ........ 11
4. General Concepts of Radiation (Basic Physics) ........ 17
5. Basic Interactions of X-rays with Matter ........ 21
6. X-ray Tube ........ 25
7. X-ray Tube Rating Chart ........ 35
8. The Physics of X-ray Production ........ 39
9. Diagnostic X-ray Equipments and Accessories ........ 43
10. X-ray Machine Accessories ........ 49
11. Set up of an X-ray (Radiology) Section ........ 57
12. Handling, Viewing and Interpretation of X-ray ........ 61
13. Radiographic Exposure Factors/Variables ........ 63
14. Radiographic Detail, Density and Contrast ........ 69
15. Radiographic Technique Chart ........ 73
16. X-ray Film and Accessories ........ 77
17. Film Processing ........ 85
18. Radiographic Technical Error and Artifacts ........ 97

19. Significant Radiographic Findings of Important Pathological Conditions ........ 101

20. Contrast Agents and Special Radiography ........ 111

21. Radiography of Exotic Animals and Birds ........ 127

22. Advance Diagnostic Imaging Tools and Techniques ........ 129

23. Principles of Radiation Therapy ........ 159

24. Radiation Hazards and Safety ........ 165

25. *Glossary* ........ 175

26. *Exercise: Review Questions* ........ 213

27. *Check Your Answers* ........ 229

28. *References/Selected Readings* ........ 241

29. *Appendix* ........ 243

## Chapter - 1

# Introduction to Radiology and Historical Perspective

- **Radiology (Roentgenology):** the science, which deals with diagnostic (radio-diagnosis) and therapeutic applications (radiotherapy) of radiant energy particularly of X-rays.
- **Veterinary radiology:** the science, which deals with the uses of radiant energy for diagnostic (radio-diagnosis) and therapeutic applications (radiotherapy) in domestic, zoo, laboratory, exotic animals and birds.
- **Veterinary radiologist:** a qualified person in radio-diagnosis and radiotherapy.
- **Radiography:** is the making of film records (radiographs) of internal structures of the body by passing X-rays through the body to act on specially sensitized film.
- **Radiograph (Roentgenogram/ skiagram/ X-ray picture):** is the photographic record of the extend of penetrability of X-rays through the exposed tissue parts. Radiographs are parts of the legal medico-veterinary record and must be correctly identified and carefully labeled.
- **Radiographer/ skiagrapher:** a trained person to operate X-ray machine in a specified safe manner to obtain quality radiographs for the use by the radiologist.

- **Diagnostic imaging:** refers to technologies that doctors use to look inside the body of the patient for clues about any disease condition. A variety of machine and techniques can create pictures of the structures and activities inside the patient body. X-rays, ultrasound scan, computed tomography scan and magnetic resonance imaging scan are types of diagnostic imaging.
- **Conventional film-screen radiography:** is the traditional method of producing radiographic images in which the exposed film undergoes wet-processing. The primary components of film-screen radiography include the X-ray cassette, intensifying screens, radiographic film and film processing.
- **Digital radiography (DR):** is a technique of electronic capture of an X-ray exposure in a device that converts the X-rays to a digital signal, which is then represented on a viewing monitor for diagnosis.
- **Computed radiography (CR):** is a digital radiography that records radiographic images on photostimulable phosphor plates instead of film/screen image receptors. The acquired image data are converted to electronic signals and digitized so they can be stored and manipulated by a computer and displayed on a high-resolution monitor or recorded on film by using a laser printer. The final digital image can then be viewed and manipulated using computer software.
- **Contrast radiography:** is an X-ray procedure that uses a special substance (contrast agents) to highlight tissues and organs that would not be visible otherwise.
- **Serial radiography:** is the making of several exposures of a particular area at arbitrary intervals.
- **Spot-film radiography:** is the making of localized instantaneous radiographic exposures during fluoroscopy.
- **Stress radiography:** radiography on structure at positioning to intentionally place stress being radiographed; most commonly used in the diagnosis of spinal disorders such as atlantoaxial instability, lumbosacral instability, joint deformity, wobbler syndrome *etc.*

- **Autoradiography:** a technique that uses X-ray film to visualize radioactivity labeled molecules of fragments of molecules, used in analyzing length and number of DNA fragments after they are separated by get electrophoresis. In autoradiography the specimen itself is the source of the radiation, which originates from radioactive material incorporated into it. The recording medium which makes visible the resultant image is usually, though not always photographic emulsion. For classical X-rays, the specimen to be examined is placed between the source of radiation and the film, and the absorption and scattering of radiation by the specimen produces its image on the film.
- **Real-time radiography/ radioscopy (RTR):** is a nondestructive test (NDT) method whereby an image is produced electronically, rather than on film, so that very little lag time occurs between the item being exposed to radiation and the resulting image.
- **X-rays:** a special type of electromagnetic radiation which has high energy, extremely short wavelength, no mass or charge and travels at the speed of light. X-rays representing small packets of energy called Quanta or Photons.

## Historical Perspectives

Imaging of internal body structures has revolutionized the modern diagnostic methods in both human and veterinary fields. Invention of X-rays made a breakthrough in examination of body tissues in human medicine in the previous century. This soon caught up in veterinary medicine too.

More than 100 years have passed since the discovery of X-rays on November 8, 1895 and many advances have been added in imaging modalities, still conventional radiography continue to be the major diagnostic modality in veterinary practice in most of the part of the country. Public fancy was caught by this invisible ray with the ability to pass through solid matter and in conjunction with a photographic plate, provide a picture of bones and interior body parts. Scientific fancy was captured by the demonstration of a wavelength shorter than light. This generated new possibilities in physics, and for investigating the structure of matter. Much enthusiasm was generated about potential applications of rays as an aid in medicine and surgery. Within a month after the announcement of the discovery, several medical radiographs had been made in Europe and the United States, which were used by surgeons to guide them in their work.

- In around 1875, X-rays were found emanating from Crookes tubes/ experimental discharge tubes invented by scientists investigating the cathode rays (energetic electron beams), that were first created in the Crookes tubes.
- In 1877, Pulyui (Ukrainian-born), a lecturer in experimental physics at the University of Vienna, constructed various designs of vacuum discharge tube to investigate their properties.
- In April 1887, Nokola Tesla began to investigate X-rays using high voltages and tubes of his own design, as well as Crookes tubes.
- In 1824–1914, German physicist Johann Hittorf and early researcher of the Crookes tube found when he placed unexposed photographic plates near the tube, that some of them were flawed by shadows, though he did not investigate this effect.
- By 1892, Tesla generalized the phenomenon as radiant energy of "invisible" kinds and performed several such experiments, but he did not categorize the emissions as what were later called X-rays.
- On November 8, 1895, Wilhem Conrad Roentgen accidentally discovered X-rays while working on Crooks tube. Roentgen referred to the radiation as "X", to indicate that it was an unknown type of radiation.
- On December 10, 1901, Roentgen received the first Nobel Prize in Physics for discovery of X-rays. This single discovery revolutionized the entire medical field and developed into a separate discipline. Roentgen discovered its medical use when he made a picture of his wife's hand which clearly revealed her wedding ring and her bones on a photographic plate formed due to X-rays. The photograph of his wife's hand was the first ever photograph of a human body part using X-rays. When she saw the picture, she said "I have seen my death". The many applications of X-rays immediately generated enormous interest. Workshops began making specialized versions of Crookes tubes for generating X-rays.

- In 1895, Thomas Edison investigated materials ability to fluorescence when exposed to X-rays, and found that calcium tungstate was the most effective substance. Around March 1896, the fluoroscope he developed became the standard for medical X-ray examinations.
- On 11 January 1896, the first use of X-rays under clinical conditions was by John Hall-Edwards in Birmingham, England, when he radiographed a needle stuck in the hand of an associate.
- On 14 February 1896, Hall-Edwards were also the first to use X-rays in a surgical operation.
- In June 1896, only 6 months after Roentgen announced his discovery, X-rays were being used by battlefield physicians to locate bullets in wounded soldiers.
- In 1896, first veterinary radiograph of an equine foot published by Paton and Duncan
- In 1896, first intensifying screen made by Pupin.
- In 1904, John Ambrose Fleming invented the thermionic diode, the first kind of a vacuum tube.
- In about 1906, the physicist Charles Barkla discovered that X-rays could be scattered by gases, and that each element had a characteristic X-ray. He won the 1917 Nobel Prize in Physics for this discovery.
- In 1906-1912, R. Eberlein (Berlin) was first to report radiation therapy in veterinary practice.
- In 1912, Max von Laue, Paul Knipping, and Walter Friedrich first observed the diffraction of X-rays by crystals. This discovery, along with the early work of Paul Peter Ewald, William Henry Bragg, and William Lawrence Bragg, gave birth to the field of X-ray crystallography.
- In 1913, William D. Coolidge (USA) invented the Coolidge tube which permitted continuous production of X-rays, this type of tube is still in use today.
- In 1913, Gustav Bucky invented grid to remove scatter radiation.
- In 1913 Kodak introduced first prepackaged X-ray film.
- In 1914, start of X-ray tube development.

- In 1915, Gustav Bucky developed the grid to eliminate scatter radiation, which later became known as Bucky diaphragm.
- In 1919, Moving grid invented by Dr. Hollis Potter and was known as the Potter-Bucky diaphragm.
- In 1921 first machine made X-ray packet was introduced.
- In 1928, first international recommendations on radiation safety precautions were published.
- In 1945, Gray Schnelle wrote first American book on Veterinary Radiology.
- In 1950, the X-ray microscope was developed.
- In early 1954, X-ray image intensifier and medical application of ultrasound.
- In 1954, American Veterinary Radiological Society (AVRS) held its first meeting and W. D. Carlson took a leading role to develop veterinary radiology in USA.
- In 1960, first radiographic film with polyester base was developed.
- In 1960, American Board of Veterinary Radiologists (ABVR) renamed as American College of Veterinary Radiologists (ACVR) was formed and AVRS brought out its first proceedings which are now a renowed journal "Veterinary Radiology and Ultrasound".
- In 1972, Rare earth intensifying screens were invented.
- In 1972, Computerized Axial Tomography (CAT) scan developed by G.N. Hounsfield.
- In 1978, Interventional radiologist Charles Dotter, known as the "Father of Interventional Radiology" for pioneering the technique, was nominated for the Noble Prize in Physiology or Medicine.
- In 2009, the British public voted the X-ray machine the most important modern discovery.

Developments in the realm of diagnostic imaging during the past two decades have revolutionized the veterinarians ability to perform noninvasive diagnostic evaluation of their patients. Educational techniques and materials will need to be revised and updated to keep pace with technology and meet the requirements of industry. These needs may well be met with computers. Computer programs can simulate radiographic inspections using a computer aided design (CAD) model of a part to produce physically accurate simulated X-ray radiographic images. Programs allow the operator to select different parts to inspect, adjust the placement and orientation of the part to obtain the proper equipment/part relationships, and adjust all the usual X-ray generator settings to arrive at the desired radiographic film exposure. Simulators and computers may well become the primary tool for instructors as well as students in the technical classroom. Although many of the methods and techniques developed over a century ago remain in use, computers are slowly becoming a part of radiographic inspection. Radiographers of the future will capture images in digitized form and e-mail them to the customer when the inspection has been completed. Film evaluation will likely be left to computers. Systems will be able to scan a part and present a three-dimensional image to the radiographer, to locate the defect within the part.

While the efforts of the Indian veterinary profession are laudable, we still have miles to go, to match the growing client and industry expectations and need to keep pace with the growth in veterinary imaging specialties which occur in international arena. Imaging modalities like MRI, CT scan, and interventional facilities are still not within the reach of our field clients and industry and hence capacity building in those areas remains top priority for our research and educational institutions.

## Chapter - 2

# Applications of Radiography

Within a few weeks after November 8, 1895, Wilhelm Conrad Roentgen made the discovery of X-rays, they were being used in medicine and many sophisticated medical applications. This single discovery of X-rays revolutionized the entire medical field and developed into a separate discipline in the diagnostic and therapeutic applications in human beings and animals. On 10 December, 1901, Roentgen received the first Nobel Prize for Physics in recognition for discovery of X-rays. Radiography in veterinary practice may not always be used to arrive at a final diagnosis of the disorders. In the last few years, various types of X-ray scanners have been developed that allow highly detailed views of a particular section of the body. One type, known as a computerized tomography (CT) scanner, sends narrow beams of X- rays at various angles through a patient's body. The information obtained from the X-rays is processed by a computer to produce an image of a cross-section of the body. The image shows much more detail than an ordinary X-ray picture. A section of the body can be studied in three dimensions by producing a series of adjacent cross-sectional images. Nevertheless, radiography remains a valuable modality in diagnostic purposes and has significantly extended the usefulness in medicine and research.

A common application of radiography in veterinary practice includes:

- As a diagnostic tools.
- To select methods/techniques of treatment *e.g.* for the fracture repair, in osteomedullography to evaluate bone healing.

- To halt the growth of cells and used to destroy benign and malignant tumors.
- To detect diseases of the teeth.
- To screen normal animals for morphological evaluation in an attempt to eradicate inherited diseases by selective breeding.
- Used in the treatment of leukemia and bursitis.
- To determine the age of the animals.
- To monitor efficacy of the treatment.
- To examine postmortem material.
- As teaching aid in the subject of anatomy.
- For non-destructive examination of archaeological specimens of animal origin.

Other applications are in industry, at airports to check customers and baggage.

X-ray diffraction is also very important in spectroscopy and as a basis for X-ray crystallography. The diffraction of X-rays by a crystal where the wavelength of X-rays is comparable in size to the distances between atoms in most crystals is used to disperse and to determine the structure of crystals or molecules.

## Risks and Benefits of X-rays

As X-rays are a procedure that uses a radioactive component to produce the images, there is always risk involved. However this risk is very minimal due to the efforts of radiologists to reduce the amount of radioactivity being produced. Compared to the early days of X-ray technique, the amount being used is greatly reduced. Often the use of a lead apron or gloves protects the other areas of the body from exposure, as lead is a dense metal that absorbs 100% of the radiation produced. Advanced X-ray techniques reduce the area being exposed and subsequent scatter radiation and the amount being used to produce the images. The diagnostic benefits that are associated with ability of X-ray outweigh the very minimal possibility of any issues arising from an X-ray technique.

# Chapter - 3

# Principles of Radiographic Positioning

Radiographic positioning refers to placement of the body in respect to linear alignment of X-ray tube and film. Correct positioning is a most important prerequisite to obtain a diagnostic radiograph. Misinterpretations can result from inaccurate positioning. Label the film before exposure with anatomical lead markers/ X-rite tape. The anatomical markers should be placed in close proximity to the area of interest without overlying important structures. At least two exposures of the part at $90^0$ to each other should be taken to get complete anatomical information of the part.

The directional terms are based on the principle that each radiographic view should be able to indicate the direction that the central ray of the primary beam of the X-rays penetrates the body part being examined *i.e.* from the point of entrance to the point of exit. Therefore while writing down the radiographic view, directional terms of both, the point of entrance and the point of exit should be mentioned *e.g.* ventrodorsal, lateromedial, dorsopalmer *etc.*

Radiographic projections: are describes by the direction that the central ray enters and exits the part being imaged. The various directional terms/nomenclature used in radiographic work are described below (figure) with their standard abbreviations as follows:

- **Cranial (Cr):** describes the neck, trunk and tail positioned towards the head from any given point. It also describes aspects of the limbs facing head and above the tarsal and carpal joints

- **Caudal (Cd):** describes the head, neck and trunk positioned towards the tail from any given point. It also describes aspects of the limbs facing tail but proximal to carpal and tarsal joints.
- **Dorsal (D):** describes the upper aspects of the head, neck, trunk and tail, also meaning towards the back or vertebral. It replaces cranial distal to carpal and tarsal joint.
- **Ventral (V):** describes the lower aspect of the head, neck, trunk and tail. It also meaning towards lower aspect of the animal.
- **Rostral (R):** describes the parts of the head positioned towards the nares from any given point on the head.
- **Palmer (Pa):** describes the caudal forelimbs from the carpal joint distally.
- **Planter (Pl):** describes the caudal in hind limbs from tarsal joint distally.
- **Lateral (L):** describes any part positioned away from the median plane of body (left or right side of the body).
- **Medial (M):** describes any part positioned towards the median plane of body.
- **Lateromedial (LM):** describes when an X-ray beam enters a limb through the lateral side and exits on the medial side.
- **Proximal (Pr):** it describes nearness to the point of origin of a structure.
- **Distal (Di):** it describes a point farther away from the point of origin of a structure.
- **Ventrodorsal (VD) or dorsoventral (DV):** radiographs of the head, neck, or trunk should be placed with the cranial (rostral) part of the animal pointing up and with the left side of the animal to the viewer's right.

The terms superior and inferior are also used to describe upper and lower dental arches in cases of dental radiographic views.

The anatomical terms Anterior, Posterior and volar are no longer used for radiographic directions.

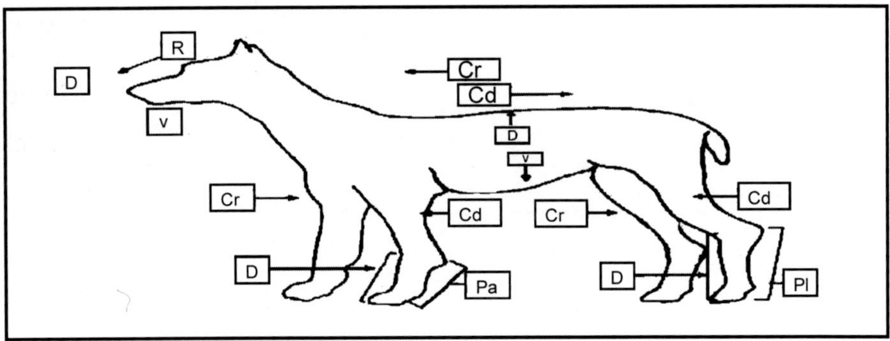


Radiographic terms consist of two parts:

a). *The prefix:* first syllable of the word often used to describe the anatomy. For example:

*Arthro-joint; Gastro:* Gastrointestinal tract; Cyst-bladder; Uro-urinary etc.

b). *The suffix:* last syllable (s) of the word, often used to describe the procedure. For example:

*Gram:* means a recording, example: Cystogram: a radiograph of the bladder; Urogram: a radiograph of the urinary system; Myelography: a radiograph of the spinal cord.

*Graphy:* means method used to make a recording, example: Cystography: radiography of the bladder; Urography: radiography of the urinary system, Myelography: radiography of the spinal cord.

**Positioning in Small animal**

| Part | Positioning |
|---|---|
| **For limb** | |
| Shoulder joint | Craniocaudal (CrCd) |
| | Mediolateral (ML) |
| Humerus | Mediolateral (ML) |
| | Craniocaudal (CrCd) |
| Elbow joint | Craniocaudal (CrCd) |
| | Mediolateral (ML) |
| Radius and ulna | Craniocaudal (CrCd) |
| | Mediolateral (ML) |

*Contd.*

| | |
|---|---|
| Carpus | Dorsopalmer (DPa) |
| | Mediolateral (ML) |
| Metacarpus and phalanges | Dorsopalmer (DPa) |
| | Mediolateral (ML) |
| **Hind limb** | |
| Hip joint | Ventrodorsal (VD) |
| | Lateral (L) |
| Femur | Craniocaudal (CrCd) |
| | Mediolateral (ML) |
| Stifle joint | Craniocaudal (CrCd) |
| | Mediolateral (ML) |
| Tibia | Craniocaudal (CrCd) |
| | Mediolateral (ML) |
| Tarsus | Dorsoplanter (DPl) |
| | Mediolateral (ML) |
| Metatarsus and phalanges | Dorsoplanter (DPl) |
| | Mediolateral (ML) |
| **Spine** | |
| Cervical | Ventrodorsal (VD)Lateral (L) |
| Thoracic | Ventrodorsal (VD)Lateral (L) |
| Lumber | Ventrodorsal (VD)Lateral (L) |
| Sacrum | Ventrodorsal (VD)Lateral (L) |
| Thorax and abdomen | Ventrodorsal (VD)Lateral (L) |
| Skull | Ventrodorsal (VD)Lateral (L) |
| Teeth upper jaw | Dorsoventeral (DV) |

**Positioning in Large animal**

| Part | Positioning view |
|---|---|
| **For limb** | |
| Shoulder joint or scapula | Mediolateral (ML) |
| Humerus | Mediolateral (ML) |
| Elbow joint | Craniocaudal (CrCd) |
| | Mediolateral (ML) |
| Radius and ulna | Craniocaudal (CrCd) |
| | Lateral (L) |

*Contd.*

| | |
|---|---|
| Carpus | Dorsopalmer (DPa) |
| | Lateral (L) |
| Metacarpus and phalanges | Dorsopalmer (DPa) |
| | Lateral (L) |
| **Hind limb** | |
| Hip joint | Ventrodorsal (VD) |
| | Lateral (L) |
| Femur | Craniocaudal (CrCd) |
| | Mediolateral (ML) |
| Stifle joint | Craniocaudal (CrCd) |
| | Lateral (L) |
| Tibia | Craniocaudal (CrCd) |
| | Lateral (L) |
| Tarsus | Dorsoplanter (DPl) |
| | Lateral (L) |
| Metatarsus and phalanges | Dorsoplanter (DPl) |
| | Lateral (L) |
| **Spine** | |
| Cervical | Dorsoventral (DV) |
| | Lateral (L) |
| Thoracic | Lateral (L) |
| Lumber | Lateral (L) |
| Thorax | Lateral (L) |
| Skull | Dorsoventral (DV) |
| | Lateral (L) |
| Abdomen | Lateral (L) |

## Chapter - 4

# General Concepts of Radiation (Basic Physics)

**Structure of matter:** every structure is made up of elements. Elements can join together to make compounds. The smallest particle of a compound is a molecule. The periodic table gives details of all elements.

**Nucleus:** the center of atom containing protons and neutrons and hence almost whole mass of the atom.

**Atom:** the smallest units of matter composed of electrons are negatively charged, protons have a positive charged and neutrons are neutral. If there are more electrons atom will be negatively charged, if there are more protons it will be positively charged. The total charge of electrons is equal to protons and hence the atom is electrically neutral.

**Electrons**: fast moving negatively charged particles fill the shells or orbits surrounding the nucleus. Electrons will always occupy the innermost shell first. Electrons in the outer shell will have less energy holding them in place than the inner electrons. Electricity is generated when electrons flow through a conductor.

**Atomic number (Z):** gives the number of protons.

**Mass number (A):** describes the number of neutrons and protons in the atom.

**Shell**: moving electrons are arranged outside the nucleus in different energy levels or shells namely K, L, M N, N, O, P and Q.

There is a certain limit of the number of electrons, which can remain in a particular shell.

**Binding energy**: the energy required to remove an electron from the atom is termed as the binding energy of that electron. This energy of the electron in the shell nearer to the atom's nucleus is higher than the electron in the shell further from the nucleus because of the stronger electrostatic attractive force of the nucleus.

**Radiant energy/ radiation:** energy emitted and transferred or propagated through the matter is called radiation or radiant energy.

**Ionization**: the process of removing the electron from the atom is known as ionization, which requires energy. The energy of an X-ray is known as a photon of energy.

**Ionizing radiation**: a type of radiation that is capable of removing one or more orbital electron from an atom after interaction.

It is basically of two types: **i) Particulate or corpuscular radiations**: These radiations are composed of subatomic particles of the matter and may either be electrically charged or neutral.The energy possessed by the particles depends on their mass and speed. Alpha, and beta particles, protons, electron, neutrons, nuclear fragments belong to this group. (ii). **Electromagnetic radiations (EMR)**: These radiation are consists of both electrical and magnetic fields set up by vibrating electrons. X-rays and gamma rays are types of ionizing radiation. The changing magnetic field is perpendicular to the electric field. It does have a wave nature as well as particulate nature (sounds strange). EMR can be represented as a "sine wave" model, which is characterized by two related parameters-frequency and wavelength. The velocity of EMR, which is the speed of light, is the product of frequency and the wavelength.

Velocity (m/sec)= frequency (per sec.) × wavelength (m)

All types of EMR travel at a speed of light; thus frequency is inversely proportional to wavelength. The energy of wavelength of EMR is related to wavelength by the formula:

Energy= Planck's constant × speed light / wavelength

Thus, energy is therefore also inversely proportional to wavelength. The designated wavelengths (or frequency) of many types of EMR however, often overlap. For example, wavelength of high energy (Hard) X-rays overlaps with gamma rays and wavelength of low energy (Soft) X-rays overlap with the range of extreme ultraviolet.

## Basic Properties of X-rays

Because X-rays are widely applied yet potential harmful, their basic properties must be understood.

- X-rays can be defined as non-luminous electromagnetic radiation of low wavelength (0.1 to 0.5 $A^0$) with high energy (25-125 KeV) to excite or ionize atoms and molecules of a substance in the diagnostic X-rays range for medical application.
- Because of their high energy these rays are capable to penetrate material, which readily absorb and reflect visible light.
- X-rays do not possess charge or mass and thus unaffected by electric or magnetic field.
- X-rays travel in straight line with speed of light ($3x10^{10}$ cm/ second).
- X- rays cannot be focused by a lens like light rays.
- X-rays interact with matter, are absorbed or scattered and liberate minute heat on passing on passing through it. Thicker and denser is the material more is the absorption and scattering.
- Interaction with living tissue cause both somatic and genetic damage.
- Interactions with gases cause ionization and the gas/ air is made electrically conductive.
- X-rays react with photographic film in a similar manner to that of visible light.
- X-rays produce phosphorescence/ fluorescence in certain crystalline materials *e.g.* calcium tungstate, zinc cadmium sulphide.
- X-rays produce a latent image on photographic film, which can then be made visible by the development process.
- X rays may be diffracted by passage through a crystal or by reflection (scattering) from a crystal, which consists of regular lattices of atoms that serve as fine diffraction gratings.

## Chapter - 5

# Basic Interactions of X-rays with Matter

To understand how radiographs are produced by using X-rays, an understanding of how photons of diagnostic range can interact with matter is necessary in five possible mechanism of interaction:

- Coherent scattering.
- Photoelectric absorption.
- Compton scattering.
- Pair production.
- Photodisintegration.

However only photoelectric absorption and compton scattering are of much importance in photon energy range used in diagnostic radiology (30-150 kev), therefore only these are being discussed here.

### Coherent Scattering or Classical Scattering

- A low energy photon (<15Kev) interacts with electrons of an atom causing excitation with no reduction in energy of the incident photon and minimum change in the direction of the photon.
- No ionization of the photon.
- It is not useful in the production of the radiograph and is, in fact, disadvantageous because the scattered photons may strike the X-ray film and degrade image quality or they may

strike the radiographer, thereby increasing personnel exposure to radiation hazard.

## Photoelectric Absorption

- the energy of the photon is transferred to an inner electron of an atom. The electron is ejected from the atom with a kinetic energy that equals the energy of the incident photon minus the binding energy that is required to dislodge the electron (photoelectron) from an inner shell of a tissue atom.
- the incoming X-ray is completely absorbed. Electrons in shells near the nucleus are tightly bound and have less kinetic energy than those in peripheral shells. Electrons of the most peripheral shell are essentially "free" because of their weak attraction to the positively charged nucleus. Therefore, as a photoelectron is ejected from the K shell, replacement electrons must give up energy before they can occupy the shell. This energy is released in the form of a photon, called a characteristic radiation because shell energy levels are specific to the type of the atom. In tissue, the energy of such radiation is extremely low and is absorbed.

## Compton / Incoherent Scattering

- an X-ray produced in the X-ray tube ejects an electron, usually from an outer shell, of a tissue atom. The incoming photon is scattered, not absorbed as in photoelectric process, but it has lower energy.
- the electron recoil (Compton) at a specific angle and the photon scatters at another specific angle. The ejected electron and scattered photon may continue and produce additional ionizations. Compton scatter produces most of the radiation fog in diagnostic radiology and is a major hazard especially during fluoroscopy.

## Attenuation of X-rays

- Attenuation is the reduction in intensity of an X-ray beam as it passes through an object due to the absorption and scattering of photons. Or the combination of scatter and absorption of X-rays is known as attenuation. (attenuation =

scatter + absorption). This is made up of the absorption of the beam within the patient and the amount of scatter.

- The amount of attenuation that occurs depends on the intensity of the original X-ray beam and the physical properties of the object through which the X-ray beam passes.

Following factors affect the attenuation:

a) Energy of radiation (intensity of incident beam): higher the energy, lesser the attenuation.

b) Atomic number of the absorber: generally at lower kVp range attenuation increases as the effective atomic number of absorber increases.

c) Thickness of the absorber: a constant number of photons are absorbed per centimeter of thickness so it is directly proportional to the thickness.

d) Density of the absorber (density refers to the quantity of matter per unit volume): density, in general is directly related to atomic number of the tissue, hence attenuation is directly proportional to the density also.

# Chapter - 6

# X-ray Tube

- An X-ray tube is an energy converter. It receives electrical energy and converts it into two other forms: X-radiation and heat.
- It is a source of X-rays used in diagnostic radiology.
- Designed and constructed to maximize X-ray production and to dissipate heat as rapidly as possible.
- It is a thermo ionic diode type electronic vacuum tube where X-rays are produced.
- A basic element of an X-ray tube (Figure) consists of the cathode, anode, glass tube and tube housing.

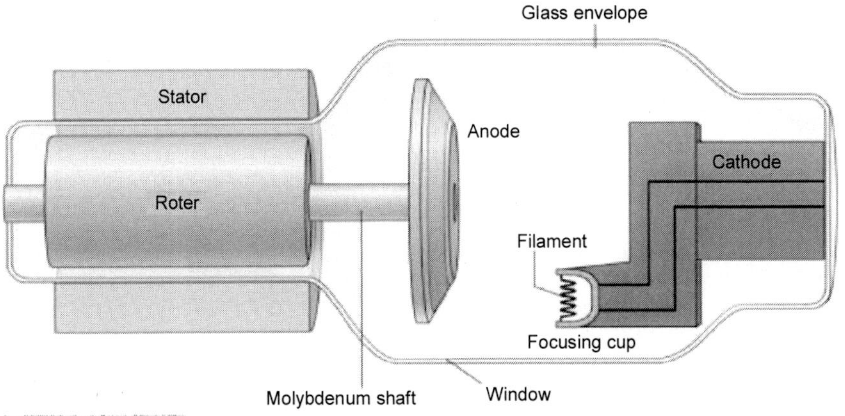


X-ray tube

## Cathode {Negative (-) Electrode}

- It is the negative terminal of X-ray tube. Its assembly consists of a filament, connecting/ Supporting (connected within X-ray circuitry) and focusing cup.
- The terms cathode and filament are often used interchangeable.
- Comprised of Tungsten filament is chosen for use in X-ray tube for the following reasons:
  a) It has a high melting/boiling point (3370°C) which allows the filament to withstand higher tube life. 1-2% Thorium, Rhenium (3,170°C), Molybdenum (2,620°C)
  b) Added to increase tube life.
  c) It has little tendency to vaporize and therefore, prolongs the life of the X-ray tube.
  d) It has high atomic number (74) which provides higher source of electron emission (thermionic emission).
  e) It has high thermal conductivity.
  f) It can be drawn into a thin (0.2 mm diameter) wire that is quite strong.
- Electrons (e-) are formed at the cathode through the heating of the filament wire.
- The number of electrons produced will depend on the milliamperes (mA) applied. The higher the mA, the hotter the cathode becomes and therefore the more electrons produced. The electrons are collected in the focusing cup. A potential difference is applied between the anode and cathode. The electrons are accelerated towards the anode. As electrons collide with the anode they are converted to heat (99%) and X-rays (1%).

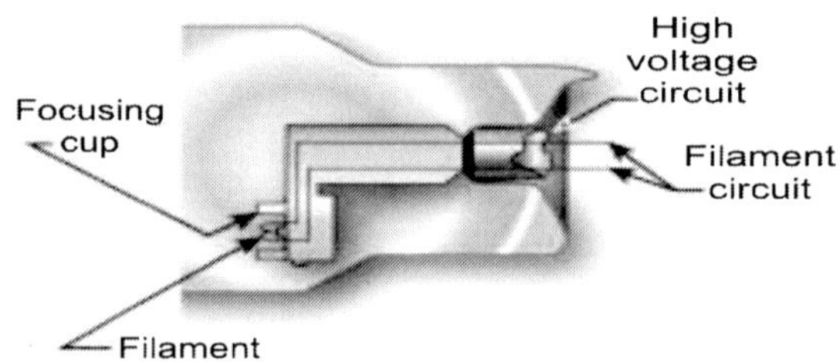


Assembly of cathode

## Anode {Positive (+) Electrode}

- Anode has a positively charged also known as target.
- The Anode is the part of the X-ray tube where accelerated electrons move to after kV is applied to the tube.
- Made of tungsten-rhenium alloy embedded in copper with molybdenum- graphite stem in which interaction take place to produce X-rays.
- X-rays are produce at the anode as the electrons strike the target. 99% of the energy is converted to heat and 1% is converted to X-rays.
- The anode serves two main functions in an X-ray tube: a) provides mechanical support for the target and b) acts as a good thermal conductor for heat dissipation.

Anode is two types: i) Stationary and ii) Rotating.

**i) A stationary / fixed/ old anode:**

- Rests just outside of the glass tube.
- Consist of a block copper in which is embedded a small square or rectangular plate of tungsten-rhenium alloy metal, 2-3 mm thick called target.
- Designed to energize opposing pairs, in sequence, so that they induce the rotation of the rotor.
- Allowing of tungsten allows added mechanical strength, improved ability of dissipate heat and reduced roughening or crazing of the target surface. Life of the tube thus prolonged.
- It is used in dental X-ray machine, portable X-ray units and special purpose units, where high tube current and power is not required.

**ii) A rotating anode:**

- Located within the glass tube :
- The ability of the X-ray to achieve high X-ray outputs is limited by the heat generated at the anode.
- The rotating anode principle is to increase in target area by rotating the anode assembly.

- During rotation the anode constantly turns a new face to the electron beam so that heat does not concentrate at one point.
- Rotating anode is made up of molybdenum disc coated with a strips of tungsten-rhenium alloy and molybdenum stem.

- The usual speed of anode rotation varies between 3000- 3600 rpm however, anode of some high capacity X-ray tubes rotate at 8000-11500 rmp.
- When the rotor is rotating at the desired level, the X-ray exposure may be completed.
- By rotating the anode we spread the generated heat over a larger surface area allowing greater technique loads.
- Rotating anode tubes can use much higher tube currents, shorter exposure times, and focal spots as small as 0.1mm because the electrons deposit their energy over a larger target region as the anode rotates.

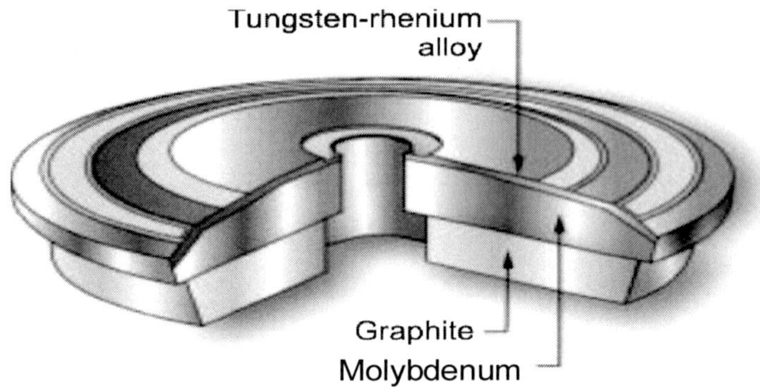


Assembly of Anode

## Anode Heel Effect

- Due to the geometry of the angled anode target, the radiation intensity is greater on the cathode side.
- Intensity of radiation is greater on cathode side of X-ray tube than on the anode side. This difference in the intensity across the X-ray beam which may be as 40%, is called heel effect.

- Therefore, while taking a radiograph of a part of unequal thickness, thicker or denser side should be positioned towards the cathode and thinner towards the anode. (To ensure even image density, place cathode over thicker part of body).
- Heel effect is more noticeable when the film and field is large, small focal film distance (FFD) or anode angle is smaller.
- As the figure below indicates the intensity of the X-ray beam is greater towards the cathode (filament) end of the tube.

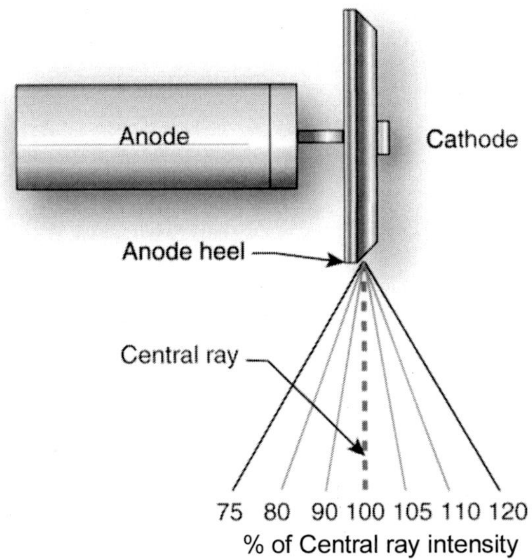


- The reason that the Heel Effect occurs is illustrated below. The letters represent interactions with electrons from the Cathode and the lines coming from the interactions is X-rays. More X-rays will be able to get out of the anode on the right side (the angle side) than on the left side because of all the material the X-rays must pass through to get out of the anode.

## Focal Spot and Target Angles

- This is where the high-voltage electrons hit the anode.
- Small area where the primary beam needs to focus on the film. The focal spot on the target surface of the anode is that area which is bombarded by the electrons from the cathode during an exposure. The size and shape of focal spot is determined by:

- The size of the filament.
- The size and shape of focusing cup.
- The positioning of the filament in the focusing cup.
- Smaller the size of focal spot, sharper is the radiographic definition. However, as the focal spot decreases in size, the heating of the target concentrate at a smaller area, which may damage the target and thereby affecting X-ray production. By employing this principle by beveling the anode (anode angle) the effective area of target can be made much smaller than the actual area of electron interaction. The lower is the anode angle; the smaller is effective focal spot size. For general radiography the target angle is usually not less than 15°.

## Focusing Cup

- The focusing cup is embedded in a concave metal shroud is the actual focal spot surrounds the cathode.
- It is usually made up of molybdenum or nickel.
- It is negatively charged and directs the electron stream toward the anode with filaments in a metal cup.
- Because of focusing cup these electrons rush towards anode in a small stream only (limits spread of electrons from filament).

## Glass Tube/Envelope

- The envelope is the glass housing that protects the tube.
- It is also used to help protect from excessive exposure to X-rays.
- The envelope is the first part of the filtration system.
- The cathode and anode are supported in a glass tube containing a vacuum.
- A layer of oil to remove heat from the tube surrounds this glass tube. As the oil heats it compresses a set of bellows, which will prevent exposure being made if the tube is too hot.
- The tube has a layer of lead that allows only useful X-rays to leave the tube.

- The tube must be completely evacuated for electron to flow freely from cathode to anode.

## Tube Housing

- The housing controls leakage and scatter radiation, isolates the high voltages, and provides a means to cool the tube.

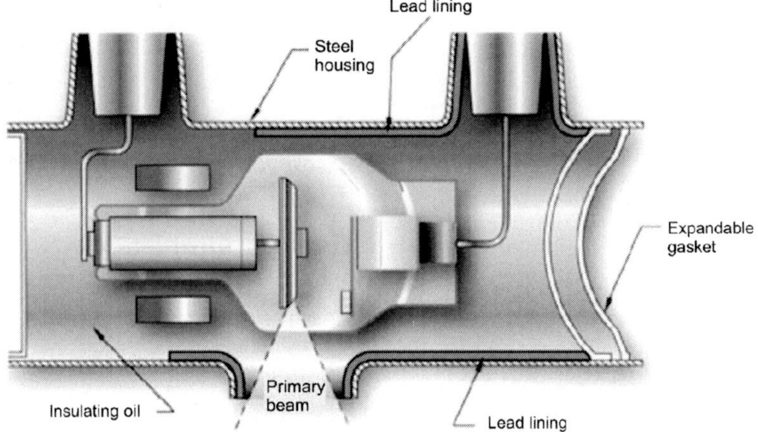


- X-ray tube is housed in a metal housing which is lined with lead except at the window.
- The protective metal housing contains sealed oil to serve as an electric insulator for high voltage cables that freed into the tube and also helps heat dissipation. Some protective housing has a fan to cool the tube.
- The tube housing also provides mechanical support to the X-ray tube protects the tube from any external damage and reduces the level of leakage radiation while useful beam passes through the window.

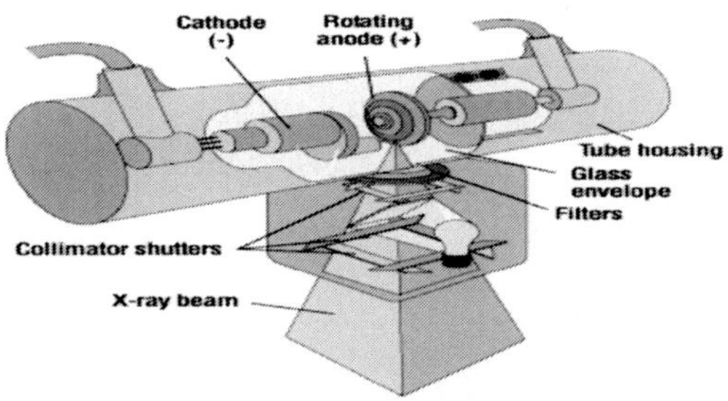


X-ray Tube Housing

## The X-ray Circuit

The circuit is actually a circulatory system for electrons. They pickup energy as the pass through the generator and transfer their energy to the X-ray tube anode.

- The generators and transformers used in radiology exist only for the purpose of providing and controlling the amount of electricity reaching the X-ray tube
- The circuit connects the tube to the source of electrical energy, that in the X-ray room is often referred to as the generator.
- The generator receives the electrical energy from the electrical power system and converts it into the appropriate form (DC, direct current) to apply to the X-ray tube.
- The generator also provides the ability to adjust certain electrical quantities that control the X-ray production process.

The three principle electrical quantities that can be adjusted are the:
kV (the voltage or electrical potential applied to the tube)
mA (the electrical current that flows through the tube)
S (duration of the exposure or exposure time, generally a fraction of a second)

The energy used by the X-ray tube to produce X-radiation is supplied by an electrical circuit as illustrated below.

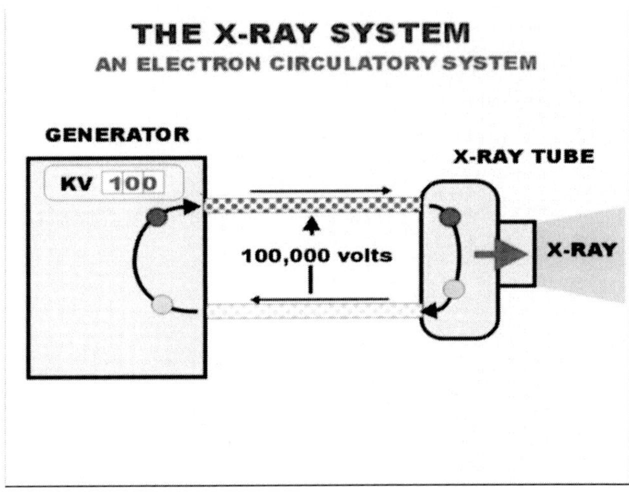


X-ray tube operating conditions
High vacuum → high voltage → high temperature
High speed → high rotation → high precision

## Causes of X-ray Tube Failure and Steps to Extend Tube Life

**Cathode failure:**

- Prolonged heating of the filament by normal current or due to repeated exposures causes evaporation of filament metal causing its progressive thinning which in turn renders it vulnerable to the break.

**Anode failure:**

- Melting of anode results due to excessive heat production by the bombardment of electrons on it.
- This damage to anode causes uncontrolled X-ray production.
- It also causes vibrations in the rotor due to imbalanced disc which increases the possibility of anode stem fracture.

**Glass envelope failure:**

- it may crack due to secondary arcing from the filament to the metal deposits on the glass wall as a result of tungsten evaporation.

**Steps to extend tube life:**

- Anode should be warmed up before actual exposure is made.
- Do not switch on ma or kVp setting while rotor is engaged (Because this causes torque force on the anode).
- Use high kVp and low ma settings to avoid overheating of anode.
- Consult correct tube rating chart to avoid overheating of anode.
- Does not run rotationary anode unnecessarily as this shorten the life of bearings.
- Adequate cooling of the tube housing must be ensured to avoid excessive heating of oil in the tube housing.
- Do not allow the overheating of the filament by repeated exposure in a short time.

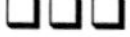

# Chapter - 7

# X-ray Tube Rating Chart

A tube rating chart is a guide regarding operational limits of the X-ray tube for single and multiple exposures and permissible heat load of the anode and the tube housing. It is an essential component for obtaining diagnostic X-ray examinations is a consistent way.

The tube rating chart provides important information on the maximum safe exposure time that can be used with specific mA and kV setting. If lower than designated exposure times are used, tube damage may occur. The size of the anode focal spot determines the rating of the tube because size controls the amount of energy it can absorbs and convert into X-rays and heat. Therefore, one should never use an X-ray chart formulated for another X-ray machine (even those made by the same manufacture) without making appropriate changes. Knowledge of three charts is important to extend tube life and includes tube rating chart, anode heat cooling chart and housing cooling chart.

To produce X-radiation, relatively large amounts of electrical energy must be transferred to the X-ray tube. Only a small fraction (typically less than 1%) of the energy deposited in the X-ray tube is converted into X-rays; most appears in the form of heat. This places a limitation on the use of X-ray apparatus. If excessive heat is produced in the X-ray tube, the temperature will rise above critical values, and the tube can be damaged. This damage can be in the form of a melted anode or a ruptured tube housing. In order to prevent this damage, the X-ray equipment operator must be aware of the quantity of heat produced and its relationship to the heat capacity of the X-ray tube. Tube rating chart provides information on allowed combinations of kVp, mA, and exposure time for a particular X-ray tube, focal spot size, anode rotation speed, and generator type (no accumulated heat on the anode).

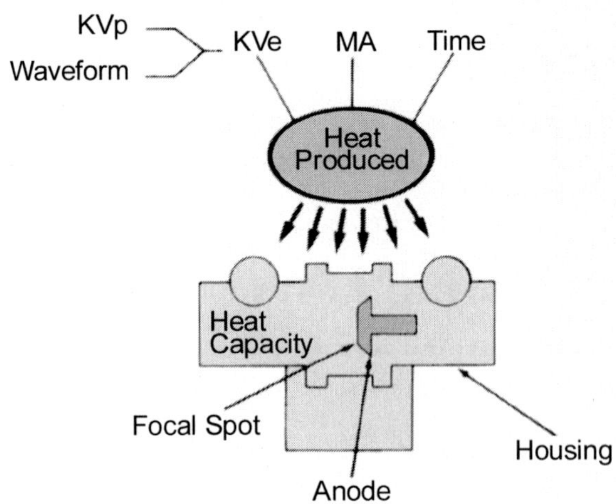


Factors that determine the amount of heat produced and the three areas of an X-ray tube that have specific heat capacities.

## 1. Radiographic Tube Rating Chart

This chart is most important and indicates maximum safe exposure time for any selected combination of kVp and mA for a single exposure time with a relatively cool tube. A series of radiographic rating charts are available for each machine which cover various modes of operation possible with that particular tube.

## 2. Anode Heat Cooling Chart or Curve

Anode heat cooling chart shows the remaining heat load of the anode versus time as the anode cools, which is not dependent on filament size or speed of rotation. It is used to determine the length of time required by the anode for complete cooling after any level of heat unit accumulated. It means the chart indicates maximum heat units that may be safely stored in the anode and also the time required for anode cooling between the exposures. After a series of exposures, total heat load accumulated on the anode is measured in heat units (HU) incident per exposure. Heat units (1 HU=0.785 watt-sec (joule) or 0.188 calories) are the product of kVp x mA x exposure time in seconds.

HU= kVp × mA × sec. × factor

HU=kVp × mAs × factor

Factor= 1.00 for single phase generator

Factor= 1.40 for constant potential generator

Factor=1.35 for three phase generator and high frequency generator.

Since more heat is generated with a three phase generator, a formula,

HU= kVp × mAs × 1.35 is used to calculate heat units.

Manufactures now supply the information regarding the maximum number of exposures per second that are possible depending on the maximum load exposure. This information is of critical importance in procedure like serial angiography.

## 3. Tube Housing Cooling Chart

Heat generated in the anode eventually transfers to the tube housing. The ability of the metal tube housing to store and dissipate heat contributes to tube life. In order to prevent tube housing damage and to permit adequate cooling of insert, the temperature of housing must be kept below $90^0$C. The housing cooling chart is almost similar to the anode cooling chart. Tube housing generally has maximum heat capacity in the range of 1-5 million HU and complete cooling after maximum heat capacity requires 1-2 hrs if an air blower has been provided in the X-ray unit.

## Chapter - 8

# The Physics of X-ray Production

X-ray photons are produced as a result of electrons hitting metal while extremely rapidly moving at high speed. This is achieved through the application of an electric current to a cathode (negative electrode) via a high voltage power source (electricity) which enables electrons to be released from the cathode into the X-ray tube. These electrons, being negatively charged, are attracted to the anode (positive electrode or target). When the electrons strike the metallic target (anode) in the tube, X-rays and heat are produced. Basically the process of producing an X-ray involves a source that produces X-rays and radiating them through a body or object, where they are absorbed at different rates until they are detected by a sensitive film or cassette. It should be mentioned at this point that most of the energy of the electrons is not converted into X-rays but is dissipated as heat. In fact 99% of the energy dissipated in the target is lost as heat, and only 1% is converted to X-ray energy.

There are two general types of X-ray procedures: radiographic and fluoroscopic examinations. Radiographic examinations, which will be used in this study, employ X-ray film and usually an X-ray tube mounted from the ceiling on a track that allows the tube to be moved in any direction. Such examinations provide the radiologist with fixed photographic images. Fluoroscopic procedures are usually conducted with an X-ray tube located under the examining table. The radiologist is provided with moving, or dynamic, images portrayed on a fluoroscopic screen or television monitor.

To produce a satisfactory X-ray, one must supply the X-ray tube with a high voltage and a sufficient electric current. The operator select the peak kilovoltage (kVp), the tube current (mA) and exposure time (s).

The kilovoltage peak refers to the maximum voltage applied to the X-ray tube across the anode-cathode gap. The kVp determine the beam quality (penetrability), which plays a role in subject contrast. X-ray voltages are measured in kilovolts peak (kVp). The term kilovolt (kV) or kiloelectron volt (keV) is a unit of energy that describes the energy of either electron or photons. One kilovolt is equal to 1000 V measure the peak voltage used for an exposure time.

The X-ray tube current (mA, milliampere) the measure of the current during an exposure emitted by the X-ray tube at a given kVp. X-ray currents are measured in milliamperes (mA), where the ampere (A) is a measure of electric current. Normal household current is a few amperes. The prefix kilo stands for 1000; the prefix milli, for 1/1000, or 0.001.

Milliampere seconds (mAs) is the unit of exposure equal to the product of the mA and time in seconds (mAs= mA x second).

The voltage and the current create the power to drive the X-ray tube to produce X-rays which then penetrate that part of the body to be examined, and imprint the X-ray film.

The heat of filament is dependent on the current beam passed through it. This current is controlled on the X-ray machine by the milliamperage (mA) control dial. The more is the mA, the more electrons will be available to interact with the target. Another way to control the number of electrons is to increase the time for which machine is operated. This is controlled by another knob on the control dial, which select the time (S). In order for interactions to take place with the target atoms, these electrons must flow towards anode (target) at very high speed. This speed is generated by applying high potential difference kilovoltage peak (kVp) between the cathode and anode. The potential voltage difference is adjusted with the kilovoltage peak (kVp) control on the X-ray control panel. Increasing kilovoltage peak (kVp) increases the voltage difference between the anode and cathode; thus electrons are accelerated to higher velocities and have greater energy when striking the anode. As soon as it is applied the stream of electron rush towards anode; this stream is called tube current (cathode rays). This enables the production of high energy X-rays. If a machine is operated at 70 kVp, each electron arrives at the target with the maximum energy of 70 keV.

## The Production of X-rays

When electron strike the anode (target), X-rays are produced by either collisional or radiative interaction, almost 99% of the kinetic energy gets converted to heat and only 1% is converted to X-rays.

X-rays are produced by two principle types of interactions of bombarding electrons emitted from the filament (cathode) and accelerated towards the anode (target) as shown below.

1. **Characteristic X-ray photon or line radiation**: An interaction with electron shells produces characteristic X-ray photons. The incoming electron ejects an inner shell electron; an X-ray photon is given off as an outer shell electron falls inward to occupy the vacancy inner shell. The type of interaction that produces **characteristic radiation**, involves a collision interaction between the high-speed electrons and the orbital electrons in the atom. The interaction can occur only if the incoming electron has a kinetic energy greater than the **binding energy** of the electron within the atom. When this condition exists, and the collision occurs, the electron is dislodged from the atom. When the orbital electron is removed, it leaves a vacancy that is filled by an electron from a higher energy level. As the filling electron moves down to fill the vacancy, it gives up energy emitted in the form of an X-ray photon. This is known as characteristic radiation because the energy of the photon is characteristic of the chemical element that serves as the anode material. In the example shown, the electron dislodges a tungsten K-shell electron, which has a binding energy of 69.5 keV. The vacancy is filled by an electron from the L shell, which has a binding energy of 10.2 keV. The characteristic X-ray photon, therefore, has energy equal to the energy difference between these two levels, or 59.3 keV.

2. **Bremsstrahlung-in a radiative or braking interactions**: The oncoming high speed electron from the cathode of an X-ray tube "brakes" and shows bends around the nucleus because the nucleus is positively charged and electron is negatively charged, the electron is attracted towards the nucleus and releases energy in the form of electromagnetic radiation called Bremsstrahlung X-ray photons. The interaction that produces the most photons is the **Bremsstrahlung process**. Bremsstrahlung is a German word for "braking radiation"

and is a good description of the process. As the electron gets slowed down and is deflected from its original course, energy is released as an X-ray photon, which may used to make an image. Usually the electron gives up only a part of its energy in the form of radiation each time it is braked so that a continuous spectrum of X-ray energy is produced. Occasionally the electrons will collide head on with the nucleus. In this type of interaction, all the energy of the electron is converted into a single X-ray photon.

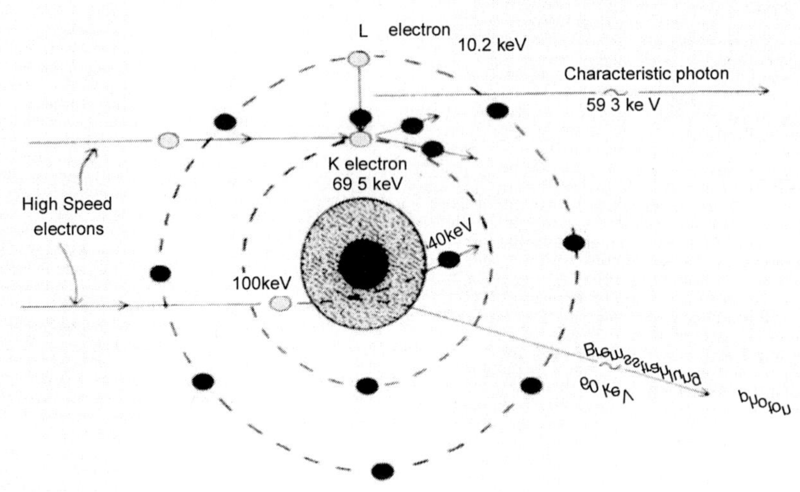


Electron-Atom interactions that produce X-Ray Photons

**Summary:**

The production of X-rays:

Filament (cathode) → mA applied → electrons produced → kV applied between cathode and anode → electrons accelerated across tube → electrons hit target (anode) → heat and X-rays produced.

## Chapter - 9

# Diagnostic X-ray Equipments and Accessories

### X-ray Machines

There are many factors to consider when choosing X-ray equipment. The need of an individual practice varies depending on the species majority and case work load.

Types of X-ray machines:

X-ray machines can be grouped into 3 categories:

### I. Portable X-ray Machine

- Is one that can be carried to the animal.
- Portable X-ray machines are widely used in veterinary practice.
- The maximum output is 15 to 35 mAs and kV ranges from 70-110 kVp.
- Cost is less and easy to move around and transport.
- Suitable for X-raying of thin and small parts (limbs below stifle and elbow of large animals and can be used taking X-rays of abdomen an skeletal systems of small animals).

### II. Mobile X-ray Machine

- Is one that can travel to the patient.

- In this type the transformer is larger to permit higher output and hence cannot be transported easily.
- They are mounted on wheels and movable on floor of radiology unit.
- The output varies from 40 - 300 mA and kV ranges from 90 - 125 kVp.

### III. Fixed X-ray Machine

- That is installed in room with proper shielding for radiography.
- This machine requires a transformer which has to be kept in the room with special electrical connection (three phase).
- Ceiling mounted telescoping tube makes the tube come across the room and to the level of the ground.
- The output ranges from 100-1000 mA and kV ranges from 120 - 200 kVp.
- These types of machines are expansive and suitable for both large and small animals.

## Operational Check (Without Patient)

At the beginning of each workday, you should activate the X-ray machine to ensure that it is working properly. This operational check is conducted without a patient in the table. In order to check the machine, you must be thoroughly familiar with its operation. Read the manufacturer's instructions carefully. Control panel includes ON/OFF switch, voltage compensator-coarse and fine, voltmeter, mA meter, X-ray switch, technic selector switch, kVp switch, bucky switch, timer switch, ready switch, Flouro mA control, X-ray pilot lamp, overload lamp, the foot switch, fuses for safety, tube head.

The steps of procedure are:

1. **Energize the control panel:** ON/OFF switch: push "ON" switch to energize the unit. Once the button is depressed the "power on" light will glow amber, indicating that the system is turned on. The X-ray unit will be ready for operation in 15 seconds after the LINE INDICATOR lamp glow. During this interval the X-ray tube and electrical circuit of the control are undergoing "warm-up".

*Note:* When X-ray unit is to be used in radiography after being " OFF" overnight or four hours or more, it is recommended that the control be turned on routinely 5 minutes before exposures are made. This will provide great consistency of radiographic results.

2. **Voltage compensator-coarse and fine:** These are to be used to adjust the incoming supply voltage at the time of using the equipment. The coarse compensator, which is having 4 usable steps of about 25 volts each, is to be used for large variations in incoming voltage. The fine compensator with 12 steps of about 2.5 volts each is to be used for small variations in voltage.

3. **Voltmeter:** There is a voltmeter with RED BAND on the dial. Voltage compensators are adjusted until the voltmeter pointer is brought on red band on the dial. Red band indicates 230 volts and it is recommended to always use the machine keeping the voltmeter needle on red band.

4. **mA meter:** This meter indicates X-ray tube current (mA) during exposure. The needle deflects during exposure and indicates tube current as per setting done on Technic selector switch.

   ***Note:*** *for exposure less than 1.5 second, duration, poibnter may not get enough time to travel upto the desired position eg. For an exposure of 100 mA, 0.10 second, mA meter pointer will not reach upto 100 mA marks.*

5. **X-ray switch:** This is a spring back push button handswitch, which must be pressed to make a radiographic exposure. It will terminate an exposure, if it is released before timer ends the exposure automatically. That an exposure being made is evidenced by the mA meter. For short exposure the pointer will merely swing up the scale.

6. **Technic selector switch:** This switch selects four technic like:

   F : for Fluoroscopy

   25 mA, 50 mA and 100 mA: for Radiography

7. **kVp switch:** This switch provides fluoroscopic and radiography Kilo voltage selections in 5 kVp steps from 45 kVp through 100 kVp.

8. **Bucky switch:** For radiography, when bucky is to be used, put bucky switch to "IN" position, otherwise it should be kept in "OUT" position.

9. **Timer switch:** This is radiographic time selector comprising of 24 positions from minimum 0.04 seconds to maximum 8 seconds.
10. **Ready switch:** This is a toggle switch of the spring-return type. When pressed, it boosts X-ray tube filament voltage from stand by to operating value determined by the setting of the technic selector.
11. **Flouro mA control:** This is variable resistor that permits continous adjustment of the fluoroscopic mill amperage up to maximum value of 3 mA. Available only in machines with fluoroscopic capability.
12. **X-ray pilot lamp:** A RED lamp indicator glows during the exposure.
13. **The foot switch:** This to initiate and terminate fluoroscopic exposures.
14. **Overload lamp:** It is a red pilot lamp. It glows when the selected factors like voltage, technic selected (mA, kVp) or timer is more than the limits specified for the unit.

    ***Note:*** *When the overload lamp goes "ON" the X-ray unit automatically becomes inoperative.*

15. **Fuses for safety:**

| Fuse no | Function | Rating | Location |
|---|---|---|---|
| F1 | Line fuse | 25 amperes | On rear of control panel |
| F2 | Filament and bucky supply | 4 amperes | |
| F3 | Timer fuse (RAD) | 2 amperes | |
| F4 | Light beam diaphragm (collimator) | 4 amperes | |
| F5 | Fluoroscopic fuse | 5 amperes | Inside the control unit |

16. **Tube head:** The tube head of X- ray consists of high voltage transformer, filament transformer and X-ray tube; all these components are immersed in the high grade transformer oil.

## Operation of the X- ray Machine for Radiography

It is assumed that before, an exposure is made, the patient will be positioned, tube head aligned, cassette loaded and placed *etc.*

1. Energize the unit. Press the "ON" switch to switch ON the unit. The unit will warm up within 15 seconds. The interval may be used for preparing the patient and for the adjusting the tube positioning *etc.*

   **Note:** *When X-ray unit is to be used in radiography after being " OFF" overnight or four hours or more, it is recommended that the control be turned on routinely five minutes before exposures are made. This will provide great consistency of radiographic results.*

2. Check Line indication on the voltmeter and adjust coarse and fine voltage compensator till the pointer is on the RED BAND of the voltmeter.
3. Determine the Technic to be used from the Technic Chart and set the technic selector to the desired position (mA selector).
4. Adjust the kVp selector for desired kVp. Check for the glow of the O/L lamp.
5. Turn the Timer Knob for the desired time of exposure.
6. Move Bucky switch to the "In" or "Out" position, as required. Placing the Bucky switch out position disconnects the Bucky interlock system and the unit makes an exposure without Bucky. With the Bucky switch "IN" the Bucky is connected into the exposure circuit.
7. Verify the selected parameters on the digital displays of control panel for their accuracy to the part for which X-ray operation is to perform.
8. To make the exposure, first press the Ready switch and then after a brief delay (1 second) press the X-ray switch. Do not release both the switches until times terminate exposure.

   **Note:** *Since X-rays are harmful, so keep the maximum safe distance from the primary beam.*

9. Switch "OFF" the unit. This step should be taken on termination of the exposure, unless another exposure is to be made on the next patient.

## Operation for Fluoroscopy

Fluoroscopy must be performed keeping the room fully darkened. No light should creep in the X-ray room for best image quality.

1. Press the "ON" switch to make the unit ON. The unit will warm up in 15 seconds.
2. Adjust coarse and/ or fine voltage compensators, if necessary, till voltmeter pointer reads on red band.
3. Turn the Technic selector to fluro (F) position.
4. Select the desired kVp for the particular patient considered the thickness of the body part to screened.
5. Press the Foot switch or the X-ray switch on the control and observe mA on the mA meter. Adjust it as per the above chart by Fluoro mA control.
6. Close all the doors/ windows of the room. Switch off all lights and darken the room.
7. Position the patient and fluoroscopy screen. Close the room and wait for eye adaptation. It is recommended by the radiation safety authorities, that the eye must be adapted for minimum 10 minutes.
8. After the screening is over, switch the OFF the unit. This step should be taken if no other exposure is to be made immediately.

# Chapter - 10

# X-ray Machine Accessories

1. **X-ray beam collimators:** Comprised of 2 independently-acting sets of adjustable lead shutters. These are the devices made of lead and are used to restrict X-ray beam up to a desire area. In diagnostic radiology they are essential for safety of the patients, and persons and also to prevent fogging of films due to unnecessary radiations. The collimator is the most effective of beam limiting devices.

   Following two types of collimators are used-

   (i) *Aperture diaphragm:* Essentially a metal disk with a hole in its center. Major disadvantage is that the aperture diaphragm allows more penumbra (blurring at the tissue interface) and off-focus radiation. This may be fixed aperture size type or adjustable variable aperture size. The aperture shape may be square or rectangular, Fixed, circular fixed, aperture diaphragm, aperture, diaphragm, rectangular adjustable, circular adjustable rectangular, aperture diaphragm, aperture diaphragm.

   (ii) *Cones and Cylinders* :As the name indicates these devices are either conical or cylindrical shaped. Lead lined cones of different sizes are available to limit the beam.

2. **X-ray beam filters:** Piece of metal (typically aluminum) located between the X-ray tube and the collimator box and in the path of the primary beam. Filters have 2.5 mm Al equivalence filtration for tubes operating above 70 kVp.

*Purpose:* to remove non-diagnostic, low-energy photons from the primary beam which in turn reduces skin dose to the patient. Filtration will reduce exposure rate and affects beam quality/energy/penetrating ability.

General recommendations for the use of filters-

0.5 mm for < 50 kVp

1.5 mm for 50-70 kVp

2.5 mm for > 70 kVp.

3. **Grids:** This is flat plate containing a series of lead foil alternative strips and radiolucent material (plastic or thin aluminum) separated by X-ray transparent spaces. Grids are located between the patient and the film.

***Purpose:*** The grid is placed between the part to be radiographed and cassette so as to absorb scatter radiation falling on the film and improve radiographic contrast image.

***Grid Ratio:*** It is the ratio between the height of lead strips and the distance in between (Grid ratio = height of lead strips / distance between strips). Therefore, this ratio represents grid's ability to absorb scatter radiation. Higher ratios mean higher absorption of scatter.

High ratio grid absorb more scatter radiation, buy require more perfect centering, higher exposure and much narrower focal range. Different grid ratios are used in diagnostic radiography such as 4:1, 8:1, 10:1 and 16:1. Higher grid ratio is recommended for higher kVp range. As grid ratio increases, mAs will need to be increased to maintain density. As grid ratio increases, contrast will increase.

***Grid Frequency (gf):*** Grid frequency indicates the number of lead strips in an inch. Most grids have frequencies in the range of 60-110 lines per inch. Grid with higher frequencies show less distinct lines on radiograph but they require higher exposure and are less effective in absorbing high energy scatter radiation.

***Grid Factor/ Bucky Factor (bf):*** As the lead strips in the grid will absorb some of the primary beam, the mAs used in the exposure will have to be increased to compensate. This is known as Grid factor.

Types of grids:

(1) **Linear grid:** Lead strips are aligned with the long axis of the grid or the long axis of the table. The main advantage of this type of grid is that X-ray tube can be angled along the length of grid without grid cut off.

(*Grid cut off:* It refers to the loss of primary radiation as a result of undesirable absorption, and images of lead strips are projected wider than those with the ordinary magnification.

(2) **Parallel grid:** Lead strips are set parallel to one another. These grids allow cut-off along the edges at shorter SIDs.

(3) **Crossed grid:** It consists of two superimposed parallel grids placed at angle to each other. It is more efficient in absorbing scatter radiation, however exposure factor are increased.

(4) **Focused grid:** Grid strips are angled progressively as they move further from the grid center in order to coincide with the shape of the beam. This may be parallel or crossed. Stationary and bucky grids use linear focused grids

(5) **Moving grid:** This grid oscillates/ moves mechanically during exposure thereby eliminating chances of appearance of any grid lines shadow over radiograph. An example is the Bucky Grid / Potter Bucky Diaphragm/ Bucky Diaphragm which is built into the X-ray table. Disadvantage include increased patient dose.

(6) **Stationary grid:** These are either built into the cassette itself or are extra items of equipment which are placed over the cassettes.

(7) **Rhombic grid:** A type of crossed grid in which grid strips are angled with respect to one another.

4. **Intensifying screens:** Intensifying screens are commonly used to convert X-rays into visible light, thereby reducing the number of X-rays necessary to produce a diagnostic quality radiograph. They may be standard or normal, fast and high speed, fine grain or high definition and rare earth screens.

The intensifying screen consists of a uniform homogenous coating of minute Calcium tungstate crystals (common in practice) mounted on a fluorescent plastic base placed inside the cassette between which the film is sandwiched. The light from the crystals is responsible for over 95% of the exposure, reducing the amount of exposure to radiation required to produce a diagnostic radiograph. Larger crystals will result in a faster screen which has less detail, whilst smaller crystals will produce a slower screen with more detail. Rare earth screens are more sensitive to X-rays, flurorencences green/blue/ultraviolet light.

5. **Screen cleaning solution:** intensifying screen should be regularly cleaned for any stain with screen cleaning solution and dust and hair should be removed with a soft brush. These screens are available in all sixes of cassettes size such as

   17" × 14", 15" × 12", 12" × 10", 10" × 8" and 12" × 6".

   ***Air Gap:*** Air gap may be used in consideration of scatter reduction over use of a grid since the space traversed by scatter radiation allows it to miss striking the image receptor. One disadvantage of air gap technique is magnification

## Positioning Kits/ Aids

1. **X-ray table:** For large animal radiography, ordinary angled iron cast table with mattress and for small animal, rectangular table fitted with lead or potter bucky diaphragm may be purchased.
2. **Aluminum filters:** Are incorporated to filter unwanted, soft and non-penetrating X-rays,
3. **Cassette:** Cassette is designed to house the X-ray film and intensifying screens in close contact. Cassettes are light proof boxes designed to hold the film and intensifying screen with good contact. Available in different size such as 17" × 14", 15" × 12", 12" × 10", 10" × 8" and 12" × 6".
4. **Cassette stand and block:** a) Rickman navicular block made up of hard wood with longitudinal wedge cut of it. b) Plain wooden blocks: 6" x6" x1" size is useful for supporting films and positioning.
5. **Sand bags:** 12" long and 3" thick and soft pads for securing the animal in position whilst the radiograph is being exposed.
6. **Cradles:** Radiolucent cradles or troughs are necessary for a variety of radiographic positions.
7. **X-ray films:** Films are available in various sizes. The standard sizes such as 17" × 14", 15" × 12", 12" × 10", 10" × 8" and 12" × 6" are used routinely. The X-ray film consists of a polyester base, coated with an emulsion of gelatine containing fine silver halide crystals.

**Personal protective equipment and clothing:** to minimize the risk of radiation reaching the operator and assistant.

1. *Protective screen:* Screen made up of lead or painted with lead with glass pan in upper 1/3rd and is held in between the X-ray plant and control panel and protect operator from radiation hazards.
2. *Mobile protecting chair:* Chair with lead screen in front of about 3′ height and comes under protective equipment.
3. *Lead aprons:* Made up of lead rubber covered with cloth, or plastic impregnated with lead lining minimum of 0.25 mm and maximum of 0.5 mm equivalent for voltage up to 100 kV. Available in different sizes and types. a) Single sides having front is covered with apron and are strapped on back of the body. b) In double sided apron is on both side and fasten at side. c) Coat type they are like coat type. They are meant for protecting body against scattered radiation.
4. *Lead gloves and sleeves:* The individuals handling the animals for X-rays should wear protective gloves made up of lead rubber having lead lining minimum of 0.33 mm and maximum of 0.5 mm equivalent for voltage up to 100 kV.
5. *Lead goggles:* For protection of the eye while using fluoroscreening against the direct and the scattered radiations having lead equivalency of 0.25-2mm.
6. *Gonad and Thyroid shields:* Available in three different sizes of large, medium and small and having lead equivalency of 0.5 mm.
7. *Personnel exposure detection meter / dosimeters:* Should be worn by all personnel involved in radiography to record any radiation to which they are exposed.

## Film Processing Accessories

1. **Film holders and hangers:** Film holders and hungers are used for holding the exposed film during processing and drying.
2. **Viewing boxes:** These boxes are used for viewing the developed X-ray film for interpretation.
3. **Film driers:** Film driers are used for drying the film after processing.
4. **Thermometers and timers:** Regular checking of the developer temperature prior to processing is essential for manual

processing. An alarmed timer will be required to monitor processing times.

5. **Heaters:** Required to keep the temperature of the processing chemical/ solution at $20^0$C in colder areas and winter season.
6. **Safe lights:** A box containing a low wattage bulb which has its light reduced by a safelight filter. Ceiling type safe light is fixed in ceiling and one in sufficient for small dark room. Wall type safe light in the wall, one near the dry bench and other near wet bench. A white frosted 7 to 15 watt, watt bulb and 4 feet away from workplace is recommended for most safelight filters. A red light bulb should never be used to replace a safelight filter, as this bulb does not filter the light; it only colors it.
7. **Viewing box or illuminator:** Is mounted on the wall to see the radiograph after processing on the wet bench.
8. **X-ray film clip:** These are ordinary stainless steel clips. X-ray films are hanged for drying.
9. **Masking / blockers and marking device:** For half film blocking and identification.
10. **Measuring tapes and calipers:** Are required to measure the size and the thickness of the part to be radiographed.
11. **Film drier:** Cabinet for drying the processed X-ray film.
12. **X-ray chemical, stirrer/mixer rod:** For proper mixing of contrast media and othr chemical.
13. **Film cutter and trimmer:** It is used to give the shape of the film.
14. **Films storage boxes:** These are light tight boxes made up of metal and painted with lead for storing unexposed films in the X-ray room.
15. **Film storage envelopes:** Available for tidy storage of X-ray films which ideally should be kept by the practice for a minimum of two years.
16. **Film identification aids:**

    *Lead markers:* are used for identification of the view and case number.

*Left (L)/Right (R) marker clips:* Made up of stainless steel, placed over the cassette to denote either the left or right view on the expose radiograph.

**Light marker:** Details are written onto the record pad and transferred to the unexposed corner of film in the darkroom, leaving in permanent mark after processing has taken place.

**Engraved plastic tiles:** Numbers or letters are engraved into the tiles and filled with a radio-opaque substance to allow permanent marking of the exposed radiograph.

## Chapter - 11

# Set up of an X-ray (Radiology) Section

To set up of an X–ray (radiology) section following points should be considered while planning:

1. Anticipated present work load (number of cases and species of animals to be X-rayed) and future requirement in the next 10-15 years.
2. Financial resources available.
3. Type of equipment to be installed for radiographic work.
4. Requirement of radiation safety enforcing agencies *e.g.* of Bhaba Atomic Research Centre, Mumbai.

The overall set up of radiology section should consider the following requirements:

1. Location and space
2. Buildings
3. Instrumentation
4. Staff

1. *Location and space:* Radiology section should be located near the clinic and operation theater so that the patient to be radiographed can be easily being brought. The construction site for installation of an X-ray unit should be in such a place where unwanted persons might have not acess. This will avoid unnecessary radiation exposure/ hazards.

2. *Building:* An X-ray section needs at least three rooms to operate smoothly *e.g.* X-ray room or radiographic, dark room and viewing or storing room.

## X-ray/Radiographic Room

For veterinary radiography, sufficient space and free mobility are the key requirement in designing large animal X-ray room. A large room (40′ x 30′) with 20′ ceiling height is suitable for this purpose. Apart from being comfortable, large space also reduce radiation exposure of personnel due to decreased scatter radiation. It is important that provision is kept for restraining devices *e.g.* travis and a casting trolly. The floor of the X-ray room should not be slippery. The wall of X-ray room should be of at least 22 cms thick concrete. The wall should be painted with radiation absorbent paint. When there is possibility of X-ray beam consistently directed horizontally, the wall should have a lead lining sandwiched between plywood. Whenever, possible X-ray operator should be in a lead shielded cabin during exposure. The room should be well ventilated but direct sunlight should be avoided as it may interfere during centering with a collimator. The building should have for adequate and continuous electric supply. The X-ray unit must also have a readily discernible indication of X-ray tube "on-off" status; shutter "open-closed" status; and an easily visible warning light labeled with the words *X-RAY ON,* or similar words.

**Dark room:** The second room is the dark room in which X-ray film is developed. There shall be a separate darkroom constructed near the X-ray examination room to save time. Dark room should have a floor area of 100 square feet. It should be equipped with standard safelight installed not lower than 1.3 m from the working bench or the processing tanks. Minimum dimension of dark room should be 2.0 m x 1.5 m. It must be far or away from any source of radiation and steam pipes and direct source of heat. It should be constructed with an air inlet and outlet with exhaust fan - these openings must be designed so that no light shall enter the darkroom while the processing is done. The dark room must be completely light proof. The door and window must closely fit into their frames and strip of belt be provided in the frame. The relative humidity in the dark room should be 40-60% and temperature be maintained at $10^0$C -$20^0$C. Dark room painting is done either good quality paint of green or white. The highest sensitivity of X-ray film is in blue region of the spectrum, so the safe light should be made with amber green or red filter. Amber filter provides the maximum visibility with minimum fogging tendency.

Dark room contains master tank, for manual processing, or an automatic processor or both. It is desirable that room should have a metallic stem dial type thermometer and mercury or alcohol thermometer with metallic casing. There are two distinct work points in the dark room: working dry bench, where the film is loaded or unloaded and wet/ sink bench where processing of the exposed X-ray film is done to obtain the radiograph. The processing film hangers and film cassettes of different sizes are kept under dry bench. The wet bench is provided with a set of four tanks which are made up of stainless steel or hard rubber. These tanks contain the chemical solution for processing of the X-ray film in definite sequence of developer, rinser, fixer-hardener and water for washing the film. These tanks are available in different sizes like 9/13/22.5 litres and above. Adjacent to these tanks, sink is provided with running tap water for washing the films. One viewing box or illuminator is mounted on the wall to see the radiograph after processing on the wet bench.

3. *Instrumentation:* The X-ray room contains X-ray machine (Portable X-ray machine, Mobile X-ray machine and Fixed X-ray machine). For radiography, X-ray table may be purchased with machine.

   *Control panel area:* There should be a protective partition with a lead glass window (30 cm x 30 cm) to view the animal and machine during exposure.

4. *Staff requirement:* Radiologist/radiographer is must to run an X-ray section to produce quality radiographs and correct interpretation. In teaching institute, radiology needs to be developed as discipline.

Large animal X-ray room, small animal X-ray room, dark room, film room, radiographers office and control panel area should be available as minimum room requirement for X-ray at teaching Veterinary polyclinics.

## Chapter - 12

# Handling, Viewing and Interpretation of X-ray

## Handling

X-ray film is delicate and should not be handled carelessly or roughly. Avoid touching its surfaces, holding it as near the edges as possible with clean, dry hands. It is sensitive to maltreatment of any kind; heat and light adversely affect the emulsion. It can be handled safely and rapidly for all radiographic purposes as long as the X-ray specialist uses precaution to avoid the production of foreign marks (artifacts) on the film.

Cassettes with exposed film should be opened in a dark room and the film is removed by holding the corners. The film is loaded in a suitable size cassette and stored in lead lined boxes. The loaded cassettes and the exposed film cassettes are kept with radiopaque surface upwards. Unexposed film boxes are always kept in lead lined boxes.

## Viewing

Radiography should be viewed on a good evenly lit viewing box in a semi darkened room. Dorsoventral chest, ventro dorsal abdomen or skull is viewed with a right side of the film facing the viewer's left side. Lateral view radiograhs are viewed by placing it facing left. Radiographs of extremities are viewed with lateral aspect on left side of the viewer.

## Interpretation

The three important factors to be considered before interpreting a radiograph are:

1. Case history
2. Physical examination
3. Correct radiographic technique

## Radiographic Diagnosis

Radiographic diagnosis consists of two parts namely location of the lesion and classification of the lesion. Location of the lesion requires knowledge of normal radiographic anatomy, basic radiographic signs in terms of changes such as size, architecture, contour, density, position and function. A systematic and methodical examination of each radiograph will prevent overlooking unexposed lesion.

## Classification of Lesion

The lesions in the radiograph are classified as developmental, metabolic, traumatic, infectious, neoplastic and degenerative.

# Chapter - 13

# Radiographic Exposure Factors/ Variables

The radiographic appearance of various tissues is influenced by a number of factors which determine the character of X-rays. Various exposure factors control the radiographic dentsity, detail and contrast: milliamperage (mA), time (sec), kilovoltage (kV), focal spot/film distance (FFD) and object-film distance (OFD), thickness and nature of the part radiogaphed, speed and type of film and intensifying screens, temperature and time of developing, grid type, incoming line voltage, make and type of X-ray machine. Of these, first five exposure factors (milliamperage (mA), time (sec), kilovoltage (kV), focal spot/ film distance (FFD) and object-film distance (OFD) are very important as radiographic technique chart may be worked out by varying one or more of the five factors. These exposure factors are integral to image quality and should, therefore, to be adjusted appropriately in order to achieve a diagnostic radiograph of optimal quality (image contrast, brightness and clarity).

## Milliamperage (mA)

- Is the amount of electrical current applied to filament (cathode) of the X-ray tube to produce X-rays affects number of X-rays produced, done by controlling the temperature of the cathode.
- mA setting regulates the quantity of electrons boiled off at the filament (cathode) in the X-ray tube.

- Usually combined with time (s) to enable mAs to be altered as a single setting.
- Higher mAs means greater number of X-rays will be produced and pass through the patient to reach the cassette (and vice versa).
- Alters the overall brightness of the image (overall more 'light' or 'dark').
- For example, if mAs is too low, the resultant image will appear grainy owing to inadequate numbers of X-rays reaching the cassette/plate. However, if the overall image exposure is acceptable, increasing the mAs to resolve the grainy appearance must be accompanied by a concurrent decrease in the kV in order to maintain the same level of image 'darkness'.

## Exposure Time in Seconds (s)

- The exposure time is the length of time current applied to cathode to produce X-rays during each exposure.
- The longer the exposure time, the greater the number of X-rays produced.

## mAs

- The term mAs is a product of milliamperage (A) and exposure time (s) on the single settings (mA X s= mAs).
- mAs control the quantity of X-rays produced.
- Therefore, to achieve a given number of X-rays per exposure, as mA is increased, exposure time is shortened, and vice versa.

> - mAs controls the quantity of X-rays produced.
> - The mA and time are inversely related means higher the mA, shorter the time required to maintain the desired number of X-rays produced.
> - Always use with the highest mA and fastest exposure time.

## Kilovoltage (kV)

- Is a quality factor that regulates the energy of the X-ray beam.
- Voltage applied across the X-ray generator at the time of X-ray production is known as the kV.

- Determines the penetrability of the X-ray beam.
- Increasing the kV results in increased energy of the X-rays produced and, therefore, the ability of the X-ray beam to penetrate the patient's tissues also increases.
- Higher kV means the X-rays leaving the generator will have greater energy and so will be able to pass through the patient more easily to reach the cassette (and vice versa).
- The use of higher kV settings results in increased penetration of the tissues, producing an image with lower contrast between tissue types and a more uniformly grey appearance. Conversely, lower kV techniques result in images with higher contrast, reducing the 'shades of grey' and producing a more black and white image.
- For example, when taking radiographs of the thorax - where there is high natural subject contrast (between bone, soft tissue and gas) - using a high kV technique will decrease contrast between tissue types and enhance the detail of the soft tissues of the lung fields.
- The higher kV technique also enables a lower mAs to be used, thereby reducing movement blur from breathing (caused by a shorter exposure time).

- kVp controls the quality of the X-rays produced

mAs and kVp radiographic density relationship:

mAs

Double the mAs=double the radiographic density

Halve the mAs=halve the radiographic density

kVp

Increase the kVp 20%= double the radiographic density

Decrease the kVp 16%=halve the radiographic density

## Focal Spot-Film Distance (FFD)

- The focal-film distance is the distance between the X-ray source (target) and the recording surface (film or cassette or plate).
- In veterinary radiographic procedures, 36 inches (90cm) to 40 inches (100cm). FFD is considered a good compromise between the distance and exposure factors.

- Increase/decrease in FFD requires alteration in other exposure factors (increase in FFD requires increase in mAs +/- kV and vice versa).
- As this distance increases, the intensity of the X-ray beam decreases.

> - The inverse square law states that the intensity of the X-ray beam is inversely proportional to the square of the distance from the source of the X-ray.
> - $I_1/I_2 = (d_2)^2/(d_1)^2$
> - Where I is intensity in terms of no. of X-rays/unit per area, d is distance, $I_1$ is intensity at $d_1$ and $I_2$ is intensity at $d_2$.
> - This mean if the FFD is doubled, the mAs must be increased four times to maintain radiographic density.
> - When FFD is to be changed, simple calculation given below may be made to determine the mAs:
> - $(\text{new FFD})^2/(\text{old FFD})^2$ =new mAs/old mAs

## Object-Film Distance (OFD)

- OFD is the distance between the patient and the recording surface (film or cassette or plate).
- Increase in OFD results in image blurring (penumbra) and magnification, so that this distance should be as short as possible to minimize image blurring and magnification.
- Object/area of interest (hand) farther away from 'film/ cassette' (wall) – shadow cast is magnified with blurred edges.
- Object/area of interest (hand) near to the 'film/casette' (wall) - shadow cast is of nearly equal size with sharp edges.

| Variables | Too high | Too low |
|---|---|---|
| mAs | Image too 'dark' (overexposed) | Image too 'light' (underexposed) |
| kV | Image with low contrast (too uniformly grey- difficult to distinguish individual structures) | Image with high contrast (too black and white – soft tissue may be lost) |
| FFD | Image underexposed (if other settings unchanged) | Image overexposed (if other settings unchanged) |
| OFD | Image magnification and blurring of edges | Cannot be too low |

mAs with grid= old mAs x grid factor

new mAs = old mAs x new distance $^2$ / old distance $^2$

mAs =mA x seconds(time)

the effect of the exposure is calculated using mA x time (mAs)

A radiograph exposure chart can be constructed to suit any X-ray machine. When correctly formulated it identifies reliable exposure factors (mA, kVp and exposure time) for known tissue thicknesses. Exposure charts may be kVp-variable or mAs-variable. A kVp-variable chart uses constant settings for mA and exposure time (seconds) and indicates the appropriate kVp for specific tissue thicknesses and types. The alternative, a mAs-variable chart, recommends various mAs settings for specific tissue thicknesses and types, allowing the operator to keep the kVp constant for all exposures.

Remember that increasing either mAs or kV will cause the film to be darker, therefore a correctly exposed radiograph relies on both an appropriate mAs and kV setting to be used.

## Chapter - 14

# Radiographic Detail, Density and Contrast

A diagnostic radiograph is defined as one showing the tissues adequately penetrated, sharply outlined, and the variations in tissue opacity sufficiently demonstrated. An ideal diagnostic radiograph should have excellent detail, correct density and proper scale of contrast. The sharpness of the image determines the detail or definition of an image. There are two factors in radiographic quality control, *viz:* photographic and the geometric effect. Density, contrast and detail are photographic aspects of radiographic quality. Detail and distortion are geometric aspects of radiographic quality. Because a radiograph is a two-dimensional (2-D) image of a three-dimensional (3-D) object, the appearance of a radiographic image varies with the patient's orientation in relation to the primary X-ray beam.

**Summation sign:** The summation sign results when parts of a patient or object in different planes (i.e. not in contact with each other) are superimposed. The result is a summation image representing the degree of X-ray absorption by all superimposed object.

**Silhouette sign (Border Effacement):** Occurs when two structures of the same radioopacity are in contact, leading to the inability to distinguish their margin. Conversely, if two structures of the same radiopacity are separated by a substance of a differing radiopacity, their borders can be distinguished radiographically.

**Detail:** Detail is the degree of definition of an object on a radiograph such as structures or contour lines (presence and visibility of image). If the outlines of various structures on a radiograph are not proper, the detail is poor.

Factors affecting the details of a radiograph:

1. **Focal-film distance (FFD):** A short FFD increases the magnification of the part being radiographed. Conversely, greater FFD provides better detail, however, greater distance requires more exposure time, increasing the possibility of movement. In veterinary radiographic procedures, 36 inches (90cm) to 40 inches (100cm). FFD is considered a good compromise between the distance and exposure factors.
2. **Object-film distance (OFD):** The close an object is to the film, the less magnification and distortion there will be. Greater object film distance is a cause of poor radiograph.
3. **Film screen contact:** If the X-ray film is not in direct contact with the entire surface of both intensifying screens, fluorescence of the crystals will cause a much larger reflection of the radiograph than when in the direct contact, causing a blurred image.
4. **Focal spot size:** The smaller the focal spot, the better the detail.
5. **Film/intensifying screen types:** Provides better detail than screened one; however, non-screen film needs more exposure time.
6. **Motion of the patient, cassette or X-ray tube:** Will cause loss of detail.
7. **Over exposure:** Too dark (too much exposure to X-rays), or underexposure-too light (too little exposure to X-ray)- will affect the detail of a radiograph.
8. **Errors in radiographic processing:** To obtain the best detail; the developing process must be standardized.

## Density

Radiographic density (optical density) is a measure of the degree of blackness of the film and is determined by the amount of light absorbed by an exposed X-ray film.

The Blackness of a radiograph depends on the amount of light emitted by the intensifying screen; light production is related to the number of X-rays striking the cassette and intensifying screen. Areas of the film exposed to a large number of light photons are black (radiolucent) after film processing. Conversely, areas struck by lower light photons are translucent or appear white (radiopaque).

If more X-rays reach the film, it appears blacker (black regions). Since the bone inhibits to a greater extent the passage of X-rays, the shadow appears whiter on the film. Mineral deposits are denser and thus appear whiter on a film. A fluid density lies between the whiteness of a bone and blackness of air or gas shown on an X-ray film. Soft tissue radiopacity which includes most fluids (like blood, urine, transudates, exudates, bile and cerebrospinal fluid) and tissues (like cartilage, muscle, fascia, tendons, ligaments and parenchymal organs) is having the same radiopacity. The next most radiopaque substance is bone (thus bone absorbed more X-ray), its physical density and effective atomic number are higher than those of air, fat, water and muscle. Lead and other metals have high physical density and effective atomic number, making them extremely radiopaque. Thus air is more radiolucent and metal is mostly radiopaque: air (radiolucent-black), fat, soft tissue, bone and metal (extremely radiopaque-white).

**Quantum mottle:** is a density variation seen on radiograph made using high-speed film-screen combination. X-rays are produced in small packets of energy called quanta, and only small area of the screens are are struck by each quantum that exits in the patient. If the product of mA and exposure time (mAs) is lower, fewer X-rays are generated, which means fewer quanta to expose the film. Quantum mottle is most evident on the edge of the exposure that did not penetrate the patient to expose the film. This area should be uniformly mottled, it appears as a dappled pattern.

Factors affecting the radiographic density;

1. **Subject density:** Is the weight per unit volume of different body constituents *viz.* bone is denser than muscle which is denser that fat. Density is inversely proportional to the subject density as denser the object more it absorb X-ray so that less photon reach film. Those objects which allow X-ray to readily pass through them appear blacker on the film and are radioluncent (like lungs) while those which inhibit most X-rays appear whiter and are radiopaque (like bone).

2. **Milliamperage (mA):** The density of the radiograph varies directly with milliaperage providing all other factors remain constant. Higher mA provides more X-ray and thus more density; lower mA results in less density.

3. **Exposure time:** Radiographic density varies directly with exposure time in the same manner as mA.
4. **Kilovoltage:** Increase in kVp increases density.
5. **Focal film distance:** Variations in density are inversely proportional to the square of the FFD. Thus if FFD is reduced to half of the original, density will increase by a factor of four.
6. Speed of the film and intensifying screens affect density.
7. **Grid ratio:** Higher grid ratio allows more absorption of scatter radiation to affect density.
8. **Developing time and temperature:** Overdeveloping of the film, as a result of increase in time and/or temperature of the developing leads to increase in density.

**Contrast:** Radiographic contrast is the difference in density between the image of parts or structures on the radiograph and their immediate surrounding medium or structures. Contrast is the difference between black, grays and whites.

An image with many densities like black, dark gray, light gray, white and so on is said to have "low" or "long scale" contrast. If an image has only two densities, like black and white, then contrast is "high" or "short scale". A good radiograph is expected to have a long scale contrast so that details of different structures are well visualized.

Factors affecting the radiographic contrast:

1. **Subject contrast:** Is the difference in relative densities of a particular subject. It directly influences radiographic contrast.
2. **Kilovoltage:** Radiographic contrast varies inversely with the kilovoltage. High kVp generates X-rays of shorter wavelength with higher penetration power. As a result there is little variation in the penetration of thick and thin tissue. This result in low or long scale of contrast which is usually better diagnostically. At lower kVp, lower energy X-rays are generated which pass through thin tissues but fail to penetrate thicker tissues. Thus high or short scale of contrast is obtained.
3. Secondary radiation, including scattered radiation, causes a lack of contrast.
4. **Development process:** A short development time decreases contrast. Excessively warm or old developing solution causes uniformly gray radiographs and marked lack of contrast.

# Chapter - 15

# Radiographic Technique Chart

One of the most important pieces of information in the field of X-rays is a radiographic technique chart. If one select exposure factors from a good rating chart, consistent radiographic examinations of diagnostic quality will be obtained. In addition, there will be a saving of X-ray films because waste from repeated exposures will be avoided.

There are several types of techniques chart that can be formulated, each type must be formulated with the goat of maximum potential of a particular X-ray machine. Perhaps the most popular type of technique chart used by veterinarians is a variable kilovoltage technique chart. A variable mA second chart is probably more appropriate for the most powerful X-ray machine. However, combination of variable kilovoltage and mAs technique chart is best. Such charts take into consideration the need to adopt a technique chart for different body systems, such as a thoracic and abdominal study, as well as examination involving the musculoskeletal system. The principle of how to prepare a variable kilovoltage technique chart along with an example of such a chart is given.

## Formulation of Technique Chart

A technique chart is formulated by a series of trial-and–error exposure. It is necessary, however, to standardize as many variable factors as possible before starting trial exposures. Factors such as the type of cassette and intensifying screens, type of a X-ray film, and the focal film distance must be constant and a grid should be used if available. The darkroom procedures must be standardized to include fresh solution and developing time recommended by the manufacturer based on the temperature of the solution. It is most important to understand that all these factors should be constant because the technique chart will be valid only under the conditions of formulation. If, for example, cassettes and intensifying screens in a veterinary practice are of different age or speed, the film density for a given technique will be different.

For trial exposure, a normal dog with a lateral abdominal measurement of 8 to 10 cm should be selected. A trials exposure at a setting of 65 kV at 2.5 mAs is suggested. Two exposures are made at a setting. In selecting the mAs setting, the shortest possible time of exposure for a given mAs setting is selected. The two films are then developed according to standard technique and are examined for proper "diagnostic" density. It the films are either overexposed or underexposed, a second series of exposures is made by halving or doubling the mAs setting. The films are again processed and examined for diagnostic quality. All films should be examined and compared to each other for consistent density between exposures. The best film is selected, if one of the techniques selected is completely satisfactory, a technique can be formulated starting with the factors that produced the "diagnostic" film. If, however, none of the films are totally satisfactory, a fourth series of exposure is started in which the kilovoltage setting is decreased or increased until an excellent film is obtained.

**Initial kVp setting:** To determine the kVp, modified Sante's Rule and suggest that you calculate the kVp using the following formula.

(Measured thickness in centimeters x 2) + 40 = initial kVp

*For example:* A animal measuring 15 cm thickness at the 12-13$^{th}$ rib, the initial kVp should be 70. If your X-ray machine cannot generate the exact kVp required, select the nearest available setting to the one calculated.

Technique chart for large animals (FFD- 36 to 40 inches)

| Region | kVp | mAs |
|---|---|---|
| Skull | 66-70 | 13-15 (without grid) |
| Neck | 66-70 | 13-15 |
| Thorax | 66-70 | 20-30 |
| Reticulum | 90-96 | 40-50 |
| Limbs | 50-57 | 5-10 |

Technique chart for small animals (FFD- 36 inches)

| Region | kVp | mAs |
|---|---|---|
| Skull | 55-60 | 20-25 |
| Neck | 57-60 | 20-25 |
| Thorax | 55-57 | 15-25 |
| Abdomen | 57-63 | 20-25 |
| Radius and ulna | 46-50 | 5-7 |
| Shoulder | 50-55 | 20-25 |
| Metacarpals | 46-49 | 2-4 |
| Digits | 44-46 | 2-4 |

# Chapter - 16

# X-ray Film and Accessories

The X-ray film is the major element that record the image of part exposed with X-rays. Although the situation is changing with the introduction of new technologies in recent years. The film can be exposed by the direct action of X-rays, but more commonly the X-ray energy is converted into light by intensifying screens and this light is used to expose the film. The X-ray film is somewhat similar to photographic film in its basic composition. However unlike photographic film, the light (or radiation) sensitive emulsion is usually coated on both sides of the base of X- ray film so that it can be used with intensifying screens. Because of its importance to medicine, X-ray film is manufactured with consistent uniformity and quality, which facilitates standardization of exposure and processing.

## Chemical Components of Film

X-ray film is a double-emulsion film consisting of a transparent base with adhesive sub-coating, sensitized emulsion that contains silver halide crystals, and protective coating on both surfaces (figure).

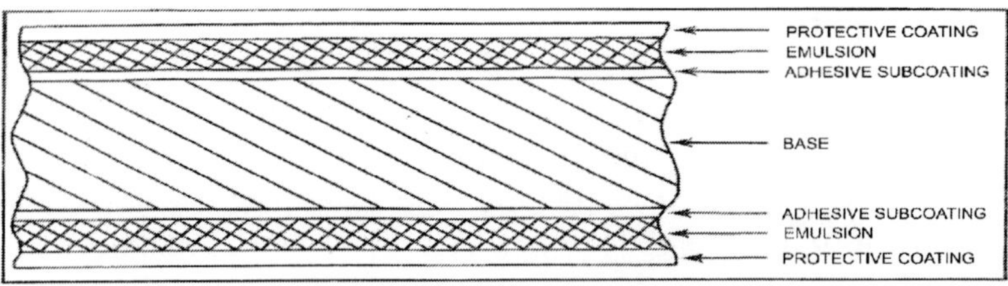


Figure : Double emulsion X-ray film (cross-section).

1. **Film base:** The central portion of the X-ray film is the base, which supports the emulsion and provides the correct degree of stiffness for handling purposes on both of its surface. Historically, photographic glass plates were used as the X-ray film base followed by cellulose nitrate in early 1920's later cellulose triacetate base was developed in 1924 to avoid the highly flammable nature of cellulose nitrate. Finally, a stronger, thinner, more dimensionally stable film base made of polyester was developed in 1960 and that has replaced all above materials for making of film base.

2. **Film emulsion:** The X-ray film emulsion is composed of two most important ingredients of small silver halide crystals (grains) in a gelatin (derived from cadaver bones) base. The gelatin serves as a matrix, which keeps the silver halide grains well, dispersed and prevents their clumping. The developing and fixing solutions can penetrate the gelatin very rapidly without changing the strength or permanence of the gelatin. Small crystal grains of silver halide (1.0 to 1.5 microns in diameter) comprise the light sensitive substance in the emulsion. These grains, known as silver-iodo- bromide, are typically between 90 and 99% silver bromide and between 1 and 10% silver iodide. Upon exposure and development, these crystals are changed into irregular clumps and strands of black metallic silver, which all together form the radiographic image.

   The atoms in the silver-iodo-bromide crystal are arranged in a cubic lattice and each crystal contains many point defects, where a silver ion is displaced and is free to move through the crystal. It is the mobility of these silver ions that contributes to the formation of the latent image. In its pure form the silver halide crystal has low photographic sensitivity. Heating it under controlled conditions with a reducing agent containing sulphur sensitizes the emulsion. This result in the production of silver sulphide at a site on the surface of the crystal referred to as a sensitivity speck. It is the sensitivity speck that traps electrons to begin formation of the latent image centers. In the process of film exposure, the energy from absorbing a photon of light is sufficient to liberate an electron from a bromide ion in the crystal. The electron travels freely through the crystal until it is trapped at a site of crystal imperfection such as a dislocation defect or a sensitivity speck composed of an AgS molecule. A free silver ion is attracted to the negative charge and combines with the charge (is reduced) to form an atom of metallic silver (which is optically black). The single atom of silver acts as an electron trap for another electron and then attracts another atom of silver, which is then reduced to metallic silver. This process continues while the exposure to light continues.

3. **Adhesive layer:** In general, the emulsion and the base do not adhere to each other. For this reason, the emulsion must be attached to the film base using a thin layer of suitable adhesive, which is generally a clear thin layer of gelatin only.

4. **Protective layer:** To protect the emulsion protect the emulsion from mechanical damage, which would be easily scratched and damaged by normal handling, a very thin outer protective coating made up of clear gelatin on both sides of the X-ray films.

## Types of X-ray Films

1. **On the basis of photosensitive emulsion layers:**

   a. *Single coated:* In such type of X-ray films the photosensitive emulsion is coated only on one surface of film base. These films are used with single intensifying screen cassette with the film placed in front of the screen, *i.e.* on the side facing the X-ray tube. These are specific purpose films used when higher spatial resolution of image is desired.

   b. *Double coated:* These are routine purpose X-ray films having photosensitive coatings on both sides of base and used with double screen cassette with the film sandwiched between the screens. Such films require lesser exposure factors and lesser processing times. For example the image can be produced in 1/2 the time required to produce an image on the single sided film.

2. **On the basis of use with intensifying screens:**

   a. *Screen films:* These films are used along with intensifying screens and are therefore ultimately exposed by light and not the X-rays. These films require lesser exposure factors and processing time for development of radiographic image. The emulsion coating of such films is also thinner. Such films are versatile and used for most general-purpose diagnostic radiography.

b. *Non-screen films:* These films are used without intensifying screens and require more exposure factors and prolonged processing time for production of comparable radiographic density to that of non-screen films. They have relatively thicker emulsion and therefore radiographic image formed on such films have excellent details. Such films are used for specific purposes such as detection of hail-line fracture or any subtle tissue change that remains unrecognized in traditional routine radiograph.

3. **On the basis of types of light sensitive emulsion coating:**

The spectral sensitivity of the film must be matched to the emission spectrum of the intensifying screen in order to increase the sensitivity of the system. The principle emission from traditionally used calcium tungstate intensifying screens is blue light. Therefore, it is imperative that the films to be used with such intensifying screens must be sensitive more towards blue light. The photographic emulsion containing silver bromide is coincidently cream coloured that absorbs ultraviolet and blue light, but reflects green and red light and therefore such films have been used without any problem with calcium tungustate intensifying screens. However many rare earth intensifying screens principally emit greener lights and therefore, X-ray films to be used with such screens should be made sensitive to greener spectrum of light as well. For this, suitable dyes are added in their photosensitive emulsion of the films. (Such green light sensitive orthochromatic films also require suitable change in X-ray darkroom safe light colour and intensity). Now a day blue light emitting rare earth intensifying screens are also available. "High lite" films from 3M companies were more or less not sensitive to room light (Particularly yellow lights) and therefore, allowed all the procedures of dark room in a yellow-lighted room. (Green light sensitive Orthochromatic films; Red light sensitive Panchromatic films).

4. **On the basis of film speed:** Film speed refers to the relative sensitivity of X-ray film to a given amount of radiation. Faster

films require lesser exposure but produce grainy images that lack definition. They also have narrow film latitude. Speed wise X-ray films may be categorized as: Standard or par speed films, Fast speed films, Ultrafast films. Standard speed films are versatile as they have wide film latitude but require greater exposure.

Film Latitude: It refers to the range of exposure factors that produce diagnostically useful range of radiographic densities.

**Handling and storage care of unexposed and exposed X-ray films:** proper handling and storage of the film ensure a good diagnostic radiograph.

1. Films should be stored in a cool (10-20$^0$C) and low humidity (40-60%) environment. Storage at high temperatures may result in film fogging.
2. Film boxes should be kept vertically without any pressure on them.
3. Films should never be stored near a source of heat, irradiation or water.
4. Films should be loaded and unloaded from a cassette on a dry and clean bench inside the dark room under a proper safe light.
5. Films should be handled delicately and any accidental splashing of processing solutions should be avoided.
6. Films should not be used after their expiry period.
7. If an X-ray film has been exposed, the cassette should immediately be transferred to the dark room or in a lead shielded box to avoid inadvertent subsequent exposures particularly in cases where serial radiography is being done.
8. The wet processed film should be kept upright in a film drier for its drying.
9. The wet films should never be touched with fingers to avoid finger marks over films.

## Intensifying Screen

These screens are fitted in X-ray cassettes and interact with X-rays to convert most of their radiant energy (>95%) in to visible light thereby, exposing the X-ray film finally with light (and not the

X-rays). The amount of light emitted by the intensifying screen is proportional to the amount of X-radiation passing through it. Generally the X-ray films are more sensitive to light rays than the X-rays and therefore the use of intensifying screens allows reduction in the exposure factors without affecting the general quality of radiograph. The use of intensifying screens has three major benefits: reduction of patient dose; reduction of tube and generator loading and reduction of patient motion artifacts.

The intensifying screen typically has following components-

1. *Base:* Provides a strong, smooth, but flexible support for the fluorescent layer. This is constructed usually from paper, cardboard or polyester with total thickness not exceeding approximately 0.18 mm. Ideal properties of an intensifying screen include: Chemically inert, moisture resistant, no discoloring with age
2. *Substratum:* It is the bonding layer between the base and the phosphor layer. It may be reflective, absorptive or transparent in nature.
3. *Phosphor (Fluorescent) Layer:* This is the "active" layer of the intensifying screen that consists of fluorescent crystals, which emit light when struck by X-radiation. Examples of typical phosphor materials include calcium tungstate and rare earth phosphors. Earlier barium lead sulphate and zinc cadmium sulphide were also used as phosphor materials.

## Rare Earth Screens

We have already noted that the interaction of diagnostic X-rays with screens occurs primarily via the photoelectric effect. The rare earth screens may have any of the following types of phosphor material-Terbium activated gadolinium oxysulphide, Terbium activated lanthanum oxysulphide, Terbium activated yttrium oxysulphide, Thulium activated lanthanum oxybromide. X-ray absorption efficiency and their light conversion ratio of rare earth screens are far superior to calcium tungustate ($CaWO_4$) type films. For example rare earth screen film combination has 12 times faster speed than par speed tungustate screen film combination and exposure is reduced by 15-50%.

1. **Super-coat:** This is a transparent external protective layer, which helps, in resisting surface abrasion. It is constructed

from cellulose acetate and has anti-static and waterproofing qualities.

2. **Fluorescence:** If the light is emitted instantaneously, that is within 10 nanoseconds, the phenomenon is called fluorescence. More particularly, in radiology, fluorescence is the term used to describe the ability of certain inorganic phosphors to emit light when excited by X-rays. The emission of light from an intensifying screen during absorption of X-rays is one example of fluorescence. However, if the emission is delayed somewhat, it is called phosphorescence (after glow).

3. **Cassettes (Film holders):** The material in the cassette box must be as little absorbing as possible. Presently, the best material for this is carbon fiber, giving a very rigid structure combined with low density and a low atomic number.

## Dental X-Ray Film

Even though most radiographers do not perform dental radiographs, Radiographers should be aware of the different sizes and types of dental film. Dental X-ray films are available in different sizes and types.

a. **Periapical Film:** The periapical film is used to radiograph the crown root and supporting structure of the teeth. It is particularly useful to determine abscesses, cysts, or granulomas located at the root apices. Additionally, periapical film has great value in diagnosing bone loss caused by periodontal disease. Full mouth periapical series are also used as a record of the progression of such diseases.

b. **Bitewing Film.** The interproximal or bitewing film is used principally to locate cavities on the interproximal surfaces of the teeth (surfaces facing other teeth). These include the crown portion of the tooth and a small area of the root. To hold the film in position, the patient's teeth close on the tab,, which is attached to the film packet.

c. **Occlusal Film.** The occlusal film is a larger film, which is placed horizontally between the occlusal (chewing) surfaces of the upper and lower teeth. The occlusal film provides a general view of the maxillary (upper jaw) and mandibular (lower jaw) arches, so it is especially useful in locating foreign bodies in the floor of the oral cavity and impacted teeth, cysts in the palate.

## Film Packet

The X-ray film packet is made of plastic or paper, depending on film size. The cover protects the film from light and moisture. The back side identifies the type of film (by colour), the number of films in the packet (also by colour), and the location of the identifying dot used for film mounting.

## Contents of Film Packet

**Black paper:** Surrounds film; protects emulsion.

**Film:** One or two films; raised dot in one corner used for film orientation.

**Lead foil:** Protects film from backscatter reduces patient exposure;strengthens packet; pattern on foil identifies when film is placed backwards (back of film faces teeth).

# Chapter - 17
# Film Processing

After the patient has been radiographed, the exposed X-ray film is processed to produce the consistent quality radiographs. Film processing can be manually, or use an automatic film processor. Manual film processing is a multi-stage process involving five basic steps in processing X-ray film:

i) Developing
ii) Rinsing
iii) Fixing
iv) Washing
v) Drying.

Mnemonic: of film processing

To remember: DRFWD (see the first letter of each component)

**Processing steps: key steps**

Film exposed to X-ray → immersing of film in developing solution for 4 -5 minutes at 18 -20°C (exposed silver halides reduced to metallic silver) → rinsing of film is carried out in simple static water or 3% glacial acetic acid for 20-30 seconds → immersion of film in fixer solution (unexposed and underdeveloped silver halides dissolved and fixes the image) for 10-15 minutes → film is washed in the running water to remove fixer solution for at least 20-30 minutes → film is kept for drying in clip for 20 - 30 minutes and dried film forms permanent image

A plan for an ideal arrangement of an X-ray film processing room (darkroom) can only serve as a guide for use in adapting available facilities in veterinary institutions. The flow of X-ray films from the exposure room, through the processing facilities, and ultimately to the viewer should be as simple, direct, and smooth as possible, involving the fewest possible steps and motions. The routine can be greatly expedited by locating the processing room within the X-ray department itself and efficiently arranging all the equipment. The actual amount of processing equipment is usually allocated to an X-ray department.

| Dimension | Height | Width | Length |
|---|---|---|---|
| Ideal dark room dimension | 7′ | 4′ | 5′ |
| Chemical tank dimension | 20" | 18" | 24" |

## Processing Tanks

Processing tanks are used for such operations as developing, rinsing, fixing, washing, and drying X-ray films. Tanks as well as mixing vessels are usually made of stainless steel. These tanks are the "wet side," and are usually used in manual processing. In automatic processing, all of the processing tanks are in a closed compressed unit, and require less maintenance than the manual tanks. The following information will generally apply to manual processing.

**Types:** There are two general types of tanks in use:

(1) *Master tank* : The master tank serves as a water jacket for holding insert tanks and usually provides space between the insert tanks for washing and rinsing. If a washing tank is available, washing will be done in it.

(2) *Insert tanks* : Insert tanks are removable containers for individual solutions, which are placed in the master tank. The stainless steel insert tanks are standardized at a five-gallon capacity. The American Standards Association gives the inside dimensions of a standard 5-gallon tank as 20-1/32 inches deep, 14-1/2 inches long, and four inches wide. To check a tank of unknown size, use the following formula:

Capacity of Tank in Gallons = Width X Length X (Depth Minus One Inch).

## Processing Chemistry

The chemistry of the solutions in automatic and manual processing is basically the same. There are a few variations between the two and these occur in the developer.

**Developer:** the developer's main function is to convert the sensitized silver halide crystals into black metallic silver. The manual developer solution is composed of four basic agents: an activator/ accelerator, reducers, a restrainer, a preservative and solvent. Each of the agents is mixed with water, which acts as a solvent to keep all the ingredients in solution.

a. **Activator/accelerator:** The activator helps to soften and swell the film's emulsion (gelatin) and provides the necessary alkaline medium to the solution so that the reducing agents can diffuse into the emulsion and attack the exposed silver bromide crystals. The activator (or alkali), usually a carbonate of hydroxide of sodium or potassium, provide an alkaline pH in the range of 9.8-11.4.

b. **Reducers:** The reducing agents change the sensitized silver halide crystals into black metallic silver.

   (1) *Reduction process :* The latent image site is a speck of silver capable of initiating development. The latent image site provides a place where the reducers accomplish the process of breaking down the silver bromide crystal to black metallic silver. The reducing agents act as electron donors to the latent image site, giving it a negative charge. Thus, the positively charged silver ions may move into the areas of the sensitivity speck and become attracted to it. As this process continues, more silver ions are attracted and deposited as atoms of silver. The final result is the breakdown of the entire crystal to black metallic silver.

   (2) *Reducing agents :* The agents commonly used are Elon™ (another trade name is Metol™) and hydroquinone. The activity of these chemicals requires their presence in an alkaline solution. Reducers are not too stable in the presence of oxygen, which they can readily absorb from the air or from the water.

c. **Restrainer:** The restrainers (potassium bromide and potassium iodide) are used to protect the unexposed silver halide crystals by preventing the reducing agents from affecting the unsensitized silver halide crystals. The restrainer limits the action of the reducing agents to the breaking up of the exposed silver bromide crystals only without attacking the unexposed crystals in the emulsion during the normal development. If the restrainer is omitted, the reducers are hyperactive and break down the unexposed crystals, fogging the film. If the film is left in the developer too long, the reducers will override the restrainer and chemical fog will result. Also, the bromide released from the crystals into the solution will gradually restrain the action of the reducing agents to a point where they no longer function efficiently. Therefore, when a replenisher solution is mixed, it should not include the restrainer.

d. **Preservative:** The preservatives (sodium sulfate and potassium sulfite) prevent the solution from rapidly oxidizing. The preservative retards the activity of the reducing agents to within controlled limits so that the "life" of the developing solution is maintained over a reasonable period of time. Since the reducing agents react quickly with oxygen, this reaction must be controlled or the developing solution will not last very long. Sodium sulfate works very well as a preservative because it retards oxidation of the reducing agents and prevents the formation of stains on the film.

**Key points in developer**

| **Component** | **Function** |
|---|---|
| Solvent | To keep all the ingredients in solution. |
| Activator | Helps to soften and swell the film's emulsion (gelatin) and ensures the solution is alkaline |
| Reducer | Change the sensitized silver halide crystals into black metallic silver. |
| Restrainer | Used to protect the unexposed silver halide crystals by preventing the reducing agents from affecting the unsensitized silver halide crystals |
| Preservative | Prevent the solution from rapidly oxidizing |

**Mnemonic of developer**

To remember :SARRP (see the first letter of each component)

## Automatic Developer Solution

Because of the increased speed and temperatures used for automatic processing, the chemicals used in the manual developer are not adequate. Therefore, although the functions of the chemicals are basically the same, some of the chemicals used are different. The automatic developer consists of five chemicals: an activator, reducers, a restrainer, a preservative, and a hardener.

a. **Activator.** The activator is the same chemical (potassium hydroxide) used in manual developer solution and it serves the same purpose. It swells and softens the emulsion so that the reducing agents can enter and act upon the silver bromide crystals. It also provides the necessary alkaline medium for the solution.

b. **Reducer :** The reducer (phenidone and hydroquinone) reduces the exposed silver bromide crystal to black metallic silver. Elon™, used in manual developing, is unpredictable above 75°F and is replaced by phenidone in automatic processors. Phenidone, which functions effectively at temperatures of 80° and 100°F, builds up the gray tones of the image. Hydroquinone, used in both manual and automatic solutions, brings out the black tones, producing contrast.

c. **Restrainer :** The restrainer (potassium bromide) is also known as the starter solution. The same chemical is used in both automatic and manual solutions. Its function remains the same, to restrain the action of the reducers on unexposed silver bromide crystals. It is not used in replenisher solutions for the reason explained above.

d. **Preservative:** The preservative is once again the same chemical with the same function as in the annual developer. It prevents rapid oxidation of the chemicals and prolongs their useful life.

e. **Hardener:** Gluteraldehyde, a hardening agent, is used in automatic system but not in manual developer. Its function is to control the swelling of the emulsion, thereby reducing film transportation problems and preventing emulsion damage during processing.

f. **Solvent:** The chemicals in both kinds of developer solutions are all dissolved in water. This is necessary both for the action of the chemicals and for the softening of the emulsion.

## Fixer Solution

The fixer removes the unchanged silver halide crystals from the film emulsion, leaving the black metallic silver. The fixer has five chemical agents: an acidifier, a clearing agent, a hardener, a preservative and solvent. All of the chemicals are mixed with water, which serves as the solvent.

a. **Acidifier:** The acidifier is acetic acid or sulfuric acid and is used to neutralize any alkaline developer remaining on the film.

b. **Clearing/fixing agent:** The clearing agent (sodium thiosulfate or ammonium thiosulfate) dissolves the residual unexposed silver bromide crystals in the emulsion without damage to the silver image. The unexposed crystals have of course, been unchanged by the developer. If the film is not properly cleared, the remaining unexposed silver bromide crystals will darken on exposure to light and obscure the radiographic image. These chemicals are commonly known as "hypo." The clearing action of hypo involves a chemical reaction between the sodium or ammonium thiosulfate and the silver bromide in the emulsion, wherein silver thiosulfate is formed and remains in solution.

c. **Hardener**: The hardening agent (platinum alum, chrome alum, or aluminum chloride) decreases the possibility of physical injury to the gelatin emulsion. A swollen emulsion is easily scratched or distorted during the washing and drying process. The hardener restrains swelling of the gelatin and hardens it so that it can withstand the normal effects of processing and shortening the drying time.

d. **Preservative:** The preservative (sodium sulfite) is used to prevent decomposition of the clearing /fixing agent by the acid with a resultant precipitation of sulfur, as long as normal developing temperatures are maintained. It assists in clearing the film and prevents the residual developer carried over in the film from oxidizing and discoloring the fixing bath.

**Key points: in fixer**

| Component | Function |
|---|---|
| Solvent | To keep all the ingredients in solution. |
| Acidifier | Used to neutralize any alkaline developer remaining on the film. |
| Clearing agent | Dissolves the residual unexposed silver bromide crystals in the emulsion without damage to the silver image. |
| Hardener | Decreases the possibility of physical injury to the gelatin emulsion |
| Preservative | Prevent the solution from rapidly oxidizing |

**Mnemonic: of fixer**

**To remember : SACHP (see the first letter of each component)**

## Dark Room Procedure

To obtain the best results from the X-ray machine the following should be observed generally:

1. Dark room should be totally dark and no light leakage should be there
2. Loading and unloading of films should be done only in dark room under standard safe light.
3. A qualified and trained radiographer should only be allowed to operate the X-ray equipment.
4. Films should be stored in dry and dark place.
5. The intensifying screens should be handled with care and wet finger marks of any chemicals should not be touch the screens.
6. The developers and fixer solution should always be covered and preferably new solutions prepared every 20 days.
7. The temperature of developer and fixer to be maintained between 25 to $30^{0}$C.
8. Solutions should be stirred with wooden sticks every time films are dipped. Separate wooden sticks, each for developer and fixer should be used.

**X-ray film processing**

1. Open the exposed cassette in dark room
2. Take out the exposed film and fix it in the hanger of suitable size.
3. Dip the film in developer. After about 15 seconds take out film from developer to visually observe the developing status. Dip it again and take out to monitor the development as frequently as possible.
4. Take out the film from developer tank after it is fully developed.
5. Dip the film in water to rinse all traces of developer on the film.
6. After proper rinsing, dip the film in fixer. Let it be dipped in fixer for 5 minutes.

7. Dip film in running water to rinse and remove all fixer from film.
8. Dry film either in open place or in film drier.

## Removal of Film from Carton

In taking the film (to be used in a cassette) from the carton, always remove the film slowly. Rapid movement can cause a build-up of static electricity. When the film is removed from its carton, it should be held vertically at the middle of the top border with the fingertips of the right hand and placed in the cassette. Careful handling will prevent many kinds of marks on the film.

## Loading and Unloading the Cassette

a. **Loading.** When loading a cassette, the film is placed in the bottom of the cassette on the front intensifying screen. The lid carrying the back screen is gently closed and locked by means of the back springs. When placing the film in the cassette, care should be exercised to avoid scraping or sliding the film over the edges of the cassettes or the surface of the screen.
b. **Unloading.** The correct procedure for removal after exposure of the X-ray film cassette it is to be sure hands are dry and not come in contact with the screens.

## Removing and Loading Dental Film

Since dental X-ray films are in sealed individual wrappings, a special procedure for removing these wrappings is required. A dental film hanger consists of a bar of metal, which is affixed to film-holding clips for insertion of exposed dental X-ray films for processing. Care should be taken not to make any finger marks on the film.

## Loading Processing Hangers with Regular Film

When an unexposed film is removed from the cassette or exposure holder, it is held vertically with the left hand at the upper left corner while a processing hanger of proper size is taken from the storage rack. The upper left corner of the film is inserted in the bottom left clip and the right film corner is inserted in the right bottom clip. The hanger is then inverted and the procedure repeated. The film is now ready to be developed, but before immersing it in the developer, the surface of the film should be checked to see that it is taut and does not bulge. If it bulges, straighten it by readjustment at the bow and clips. Since cleanliness is of utmost importance and the presence of extraneous marks or artifacts on the radiograph are objectionable, clips must be kept scrupulously clean. Using both hands to avoid kink marks, place the film carefully in the cassette. Gently close and latch the cassette.

## Immersion of Hangers in Solutions

When placing hangers loaded with film in solutions, dip them quickly and carefully. After complete immersion, raise and lower the films about two inches several times to remove air bells and completely bathe the surfaces of the film. Make sure hangers are separated by about three-fourths inch. Do not remove them entirely from the solution until you are ready for the next operation. By keeping the level of the solutions one-inch below the tops of the tanks, the crossbars of the hangers are not covered by the developer of fixer solutions. However, the crossbars should be immersed in the wash water.

## Production of the Latent Image

When the X-ray film emulsion is sensitized during manufacture, the silver bromide crystals are left in a state of suspended animation awaiting the X-ray stimulus to start them on their way to becoming a radiographic image. The potentiality for this activity exists in the tiny sensitization "specks" at the surface of the crystal. When X-ray exposure occurs, the latent image is produced. The generally accepted theory as to the nature of changes occurring in the production of the latent image is that, when the silver bromide crystals are atomically activated by exposure to X-rays (and usually, the fluorescent light of intensifying screens), electrons fly out of their normal atomic orbits and wander at random throughout the crystals. Normally, the silver bromide crystal is a nonconductor of electricity. Upon exposure to X-rays or light, however, it becomes a weak conductor and the photoelectrons, released from the individual atoms in the crystal flow within the crystal as a tiny electric current. Ultimately, some of these electrons are trapped or acquired by the "speck". A negative electrostatic field is now set up around the "speck." Other activities also occur in the crystal for the slower-moving silver ions with a positive charge travel to the negatively charged "specks" where they are neutralized to form tiny particles of atomic silver, while the bromide portions of the crystal are absorbed elsewhere. As more silver ions are neutralized, the "speck" grows with silver the silver has been reduced to metallic silver by the action of the developer.

The latent image cannot be seen or detected by ordinary physical means, but it can be changed into a visible silver image by chemical processing.

## Safety Precautions

Because of the alkaline and acid nature of the developer and fixer solutions, minor chemical irritation or burns can occur when they come in contact with the skin, the eyes, and the mouth. Use caution when stirring or mixing solutions. Always wear rubber gloves and protective eyewear or a protective face shield and an apron when working around these solutions. If the solutions come in contact with the skin, flush the area with large amounts of water. If the solutions accidentally splash into the eyes or mouth, flush with large amounts of water and immediately seek medical attention. Fixer solution can stain and discolor clothing.

## Automatic Processing

The automatic film processor mechanically transports exposed X-ray film through the developing, fixing, washing, and drying cycles. Use of automatic processors can develop film more quickly, processing and drying a film in 90 to 120 seconds. Automatic processing is quicker than manual processing, and it produces finished radiographs of uniform quality. Automatic processing is the most commonly used method of processing dental radiographs in the Navy and they can be generally classified as small or large. The large automatic processor processes all sizes of dental radiographs including intraoral, occlusal, panoramic, and 8-inch x 10-inch cephalometric films. This processor will be located in the darkroom. The X-ray film must be inserted in the processor under safelight conditions. Large automatic processors can be equipped with daylight loaders, eliminating the need for a darkroom. Operational Check Perform the operational check at the beginning of each day to ensure that the processor is in good working order. It is a complex piece of equipment, so read the manufacturer's operational manual very carefully. Never attempt to repair the components inside the processor.

## Storage of Film

X-ray film emulsion is sensitive to X-rays,ultraviolet rays, light, temperature, pressure and certain chemicals. So following precautions should be taken during storing of films:

a. Unexposed and unprocessed X-ray film should always be kept in a cool, dry place. It should never be stored in basements or near steam pipes or other sources of heat. In extremely warm climates, only small quantities of film should be ordered at one time, so that a rapid turnover takes place. High temperatures damage the emulsion, causing fog and lack of contrast. Unexposed X-ray film is not usable after a few weeks when it has been subjected to temperatures of 90° to 100°F or after a few days of 110° to 120°F. Sealed containers protect film from moisture and other contaminants as long as they are unbroken, but they do not protect against high temperatures.

b. Film must be suitably protected from the unwanted actions of X-rays or radium by lead-lined walls or chests. Film bins located in the processing room should be protected by sheet lead.

c. X-ray film must never be stored in drug rooms or other places containing fumes of any kind. Illuminating gas, formalin, ammonia, volatile oils, sewer gas, and similar substance will fog film, which is stored in an atmosphere containing them.

d. Film should never be subjected to extreme pressure such as wrinkling, bending, or rolling, because changes take place in the emulsion, which, upon development, appear as tree-like artifacts on the finished film. To avoid pressure markings, packages of unexposed film should always be stored on edge; they should never be stacked one upon another.

e. All film should be used before its expiration date.

f. Storage of unexposed packages of film in refrigerators is satisfactory provided packages are removed from 24 to 36 hours before they are to be used. This procedure is to avoid condensing moisture on the film. Open boxes of film should not be stored in refrigerators because of high humidity. Once a box of film is opened, it should be used as soon as possible. If unexposed boxes of X-ray film must be stored in refrigerators, the refrigerators should contain nothing else and some kind of dehydrator should be used to reduce the humidity.

g. Transportation of films from supply office to hospital should be done by fastest mean.

h. Boxes in which the film packages are transported should be marked "KEEP AWAY FROM IONIZING RADIATION". Customs authorities should be advised not to examine these boxes with X-ray screening.

i. Dark room should be tested from time to time against any stray radiations.

j. Unloaded cassette should always be kept closed to avoid accumulation of dust, hair or other chemicals.

## Silver Recovery

In larger veterinary practices, the silver contained within the X-ray film emulsion may be removed and recovered. When an exposed film is placed in the developer, the exposed silver halide crystals are changed to black metallic silver. Most of the silver that is not exposed to X-rays is not converted to metallic silver and accumulates within the fixer solution. Silver recovery units can be attached if the fixer solution to remove the silver by an electrolytic process. Due to this reason, used fixer solution should not be thrown away and be sold in the market to recover some cost. This, however, is only economical for the larger volume in veterinary clinics/institutions. The silver can also be recovered from exposed and non-exposed X-ray film. Silver recovery potential of 20-25 X-ray films of 14" x 17" size is about 30 gms. There are a few companies that specialize in recycling X-ray film for silver recovery.

## Chapter - 18

# Radiographic Technical Error and Artifacts

Artifacts are any unwanted radiographic densities in the form of blemishes arising from improper handling x-ray film, exposure, processing, housekeeping or setting up a technique for an examination. Artifacts will reduce the overall quality of the radiograph and in certain cases may nullify its diagnostic outcome. An idea about the possible errors is desirable in order to adopt corrective measures.

| Artifact | Causes | Correction |
|---|---|---|
| Increased film density (Too dark-black) | i. Too high mAs/ kVp setting | i. Reduce mAs/kVp |
| | ii. Too short focal film distance (FFD) | ii. Use recommended FFD |
| | iii. Equipment malfunction | iii. Recalibrate the machine |
| | iv. Over development | iv. Avoid overdevelopment |
| | v. Wrong screen/film | v. Check screen/film. |
| Decreased film density(too light-white) | 1. Too low mAs or kV setting | 1. Use proper factors(mAs/ kVp) |
| | 2. Too long focal-film distance | 2. Reduced FFD |
| | 3. Underdevelopment | 3. Correct development |
| | 4. Doubling of film in cassette | 4. Proper loading |
| | 5. Wrong screen/film | 5. Check screen/film. |
| Distorred or blurred radiograph | a). Motion of patient, cassette or machine | a). Avoid motion and secured properly |
| | b). Poor film-screen contact | b). Check screen/film. |
| | c). Poor centering of primary X-ray beam | c). Proper alignment |

*Contd.*

| | | |
|---|---|---|
| Chemical fog | Over processing | Proper processing |
| Finger marks | Improper handling | Properly handle |
| Frosty areas on film | Improper washing of film | Properly wash |
| Fogged film (overall gray appearance) | i. The film was stored in an area that was too hot or humid.<br>ii. Old or expired film. film | i. Proper storing of film<br>ii. Do not use old/expired |
| White spots | 1. Defective screens-pitted, scratched<br>2. Foreign materials (dust or grit) on surface of film<br>3. Fixer or oil on film before processing | 1. Replace screen<br>2. Handle film gently<br>3. Avoid stacking of film in fixer tank |
| Black areas/ spots/streaks | Drops of developer solution on film before processing Film stacking together in fixer | Avoid stacking of films in tank |
| Linear black marks | Film scratched before processing | Handle film more gently |
| Treelike black marks | Static electricity | Move film slowly |
| Edge of film black | Film fogged | Check for light leak cassette |
| Sharp white specks | Dirt in cassette | Clean the cassette |
| White "hair" marks | Hair in cassette | Clean the cassette |
| Air bubbles | Film not agitated when placed in developer | Agitate film in developer |
| Reticulation | i. Temperature variation during processing<br>ii. Weak fixer or lack of hardening solution | i. Maintain temperature<br>ii. Correct the solution |
| Streaks on film | i. Inadequate agitation, rinsing<br>ii. Dirty film hanger | i. Proper agitation and rinsing<br>ii. Use clean hanger |
| Brittle radiographs | A. Drying temperature too high,<br>B. drying time too long | A. Maintain temperature<br>B. Proper drying time |
| X-ray film comes out black with no image | i. X-ray film may be exposed to light accidentally.<br>ii. Too long developing time. time<br>iii. Machine not working properly | i. Avoid exposure to light<br>ii. Correct development<br>iii. Machine needs recalibration. |
| Blank film | a. Not exposed<br>b. Improper direction of central beam | a. Check exposure switch<br>b. Proper centering |

*Contd.*

| | | |
|---|---|---|
| Yellow-brown film | Insufficient washing | Wash properly and completely |
| Miscellaneous mistakes | a. Film-wet-too short drying time | a. Proper drying |
| | b. Corner marks-wet or dirty finger on hangers | b. Use Clean hanger |
| | c. Sticky films-film washed improperly | c. Proper wash |
| | d. Scratches–careless handling | d. Handle film gently |

# Chapter - 19

# Significant Radiographic Findings of Important Pathological Conditions

## Orthopaedic Radiography

Radiography as an aid to diagnosis the orthopaedic cases has become an integral part of every modern hospital. This technique may also be helpful in detecting some previously unrecognized lesions in the area radiographed.

The radiologist must be aware of the radiological anatomy of part being examined, and of its normal variation with age, species and breed. The anatomical features which can be appreciated in a radiograph are:

- The contour of the organ or structure.
- Protruberances *e.g.* great tronchanter of femur.
- Bony cortex: The compact bone which is composed in thickest and best seen in the diaphyseal region. It thins out at each to surround and blend with the cancellous bone of each epiphysis. Calcification is the deposition of calcium salts within bone which renders it radiopaque.
- The fine detail of internal structures like trabecular structure of the cancellous bone. The cancellous bone fills the epiphysis and extends into the ends of the medullary cavity.
- Outline of the medullary cavity.

- Outline of nutrient foramen.
- The epiphyseal line is sometimes spoken of as "the growth plate" and indicates the area in which the longitudinal growth of bone. It is seen as a narrow translucent line extending completely across of bone and might be mistaken for a fracture line.
- Once radiography shows that the bony structure of the epiphysis has emergd with that of metaphysic and obliterated the epiphyseal line, no further growth will occur.
- The diaphysis is the shaft of the bone and shows clearly the dense compact bone of the cortex and the outline of the meduallary cavity.
- Radiographically the non-calcified area between the bones is usually referred to as the joint space, which is largely consists of the articular cartilages and space be of uniform width.

**Indication for orthopaedic radiography includes:**

1. To rule out the displacement of the structures *e.g.*, dislocated hip.
2. To rule out in the density of the tissue *e.g.* Increased in calcification, decreased in osteolysis with bone necrosis.
3. A break or variation in the contour of the part *e.g.* A fracture or a neoplastic enlargement of an organ.
4. Variation in the detailed structure of the part or tissue *e.g.* The marked narrowing of the bony cortex which occurs in association with juvenile osteoporosis.

**Thoracic radiography:** Is one of the most performed radiographic examinations in small animal practice and for some extend in large animal. Interpretation of thoracic cavity includes: thoracic esophagus (alimentary system), lungs (respiratory system), heart (cardiovascular system) and thoracic spine (skeletal system).

Indications of thoracic radiography includes:

- To rule out esophageal abnormalities like megaesophagus, esophageal diverticulum, esophageal constriction, esophageal choke etc.
- The rule out lung disease lile bronchopneumonia, pleural effusion, chylothorax, bronchitis, tuberculosis *etc.*

- To rule out cardiac involment like cardiomegaly, traumatic reticuluperitonitis *etc.*
- Thoracic radiography is also indicated to rule out thoracic spine for spondylosis, bone lesions, fracture *etc.*

## Vertebral Scale Indexing System

Vertebral scale index is an alternative method that would anatomically justifiable, reasonably precise, simple to use and explain for quantitative assessment of different organs with the organ skeletal ratio. Emphasis was placed on comparison of organs size to vertebral length; because both are measurable in plain radiograph and good correlation are known to exist between both structures.

## Heart

- In lateral radiographic view, the cardiac long axis (L) was measured from the ventral border of the left main stem bronchus to the most distant ventral contour of the cardiac apex.
- This dimension reflects the combined size of the left atrium and left ventricle.
- The measurement was made using caliper which was then repositioned over the thoracic vertebra beginning with the cranial edge of $T_4$.
- The distant to the caudal caliper point was estimated to the nearest 0.1 vertebra (V).
- The maximal short axis (S) of the heart in the central third region, perpendicular to the long axis was recorded in the same manner starting at $T_4$.
- The short axis and long axis dimension were then added to yield a vertebral/heart sum as expression of heart size in relation to a vertebral indicator of body length (VHS= S + L).
- The overall size of the heart was thus expressed as total unit's of vertebral length to the nearest 0.1 V and termed as the vertebral heart size (VHS).
- The VHS in normal dogs is found to be average of 9.7 ± 0.5 vertebra and ranges between 8.7 to 10.7 vertebre and this value is suggestive as clinically useful limit for normal size in most of breeds.

## Liver

- In lateral radiography, liver length is measured as the length of the axis from the most cranial part of the diaphragm to the apex of liver tip. In left lateral recumbency less merging of the silhouettes of liver and spleen was noticed.
- The measured length is expressed as ratio with the vertebral length $T_{11}$.
- Normal radiographic liver length measured on right lateral views made on expiration and expressed as a ration to the length of the $11^{th}$ thoracic vertebra varied between 4.8 and 7.8.
- Normal ratio is 6.5:1, more than 7.5 suggestive of hepatomegaly and less than 5.5 is cirrhosis.

## Kidney

- The kidney size should be assessed on the ventro-dorsal radiograph because renal positioning is more constant, there by minimizing distortion.
- Normal canine kidney measures 2.5 to 3.5 times the length of the second lumbar vertebra ($L_2$), where as feline kidney ranges from 2-3 times the length of $L_2$.

## Prostate

- The normal prostate is contained within the pelvic inlet.
- The diameter in any direction should not exceed 70% of the pelvic inlet.
- Enlargement of prostate to 90% of the distant of pubis to the sacral promontory is suggestive of mass like cyst, abscess, tumour.

## Intestine

- In normal dog, Small bowel diameter should not exceed the height of the central portion of the body of the lumbar vertebra or twice the width of a rib.
- Mild distension is equal to 1.5 to 2 times of normal bowel diameter.

**Abdominal radiography:**

**Indications includes:**

Persistent vomiting, abdominal pain, haematuria, evaluation of an abdominal mass, evaluation of abdominal distension, tenesmus, jaundice, persistent diarrhea, incontinence, evaluation of external swelling.

**Patient preparation:**

- Performed a planned, elective radiographic examination of the abdomen, withhold food and water for atleast 12 hrs prior to the radiography.
- Water and dirt in the coat will produce confusing radiodensities on the films.
- A water enema prior to radiography will prove visualization of the viscera by removing the confusing shadows of colonic contents. This is especially important in investigating the bladder, performing infusion urography or proceeding to a barium enema.

| Conditions | Significant Radiographic findings/ signs |
|---|---|
| **Radiological pathology of bones and joints** | |
| Bone diseases | Altered contour of the bone |
| | Altered size of the bone |
| | Decreased bone density |
| | Change in trabecular patten |
| Joint diseases | Widening or narrowing of the joint space |
| | Cystic changes |
| | Swollen joint capsule-soft tissue swelling |
| Osteoporosis | Diminished density of the bone |
| Hip dysplasia in small animals | Bony exostosis, new bone formation involving acetabulum-thickened disorganized appreance of the femoral neck- remodeling and flattning of the femoral head |
| Hip dislocation | Abnormal width of the intra articular space |
| Long bone fracture | Characterized by disruption of the continuity of a bone |
| Normal fracture healing | Bone resorption along the fracture edges (5 -10 days) |
| | Fracture line more prominent |
| | Calcified periosteal callus first appears as a point, hazy area of increased densiy |

*Contd.*

| | |
|---|---|
| | Eventually callus becomes longer and more dense |
| | Reforming of the normal trabecular pattern obscuring the fracture line and remodeling and restoration of the medullary cavity and cortex |
| Delayed fracture healing | Slow build up of periosteal callus |
| | Failure of callus to bridge the fracture site |
| | A sequestrum may be present |
| Non-union of fracture | Smoothness of the fragment ends |
| | Bone ends attain "elephant foot" appearance |
| | Non-bridging periosteal callus |
| | Infection will cause lytic changes |
| Osteomyelitis | Both bone lysis and production seen, |
| | usually are equal in degree |
| | Sequestra are equal in degree |
| Osteosarcoma (primary bone tumour) | Indistinct production of new bone at the site, with ill defined increase or decrease in bone density |
| | Apprearance of neoplastic bone spicules-"sunburst" appearance. |
| Arthrosis | Swelling of joint capsule |
| Infectious arthritis | Thickening of synovial membrane |
| | Distension of joint capsule |
| | Slight widening of joint space |
| **Radiological pathology of skull** | |
| Nutritional osteodystrophy | Lamina dura is not seen due to improper osteoid formation. |
| | -advanced cases-evidence of bony demineralisation |
| Mandibular periostitis | Sclerosis and active new bone production at the tympanic bulla |
| Skull fractures | -Occult fractures-associated with soft tissue swelling |
| | -discontinuity of bony structure |
| Temporal mandibular luxation | Displacement of mandibular condyles away from the post glenoid process in VD projection |
| Neoplasia | Osteoma: rounded sclerotic, smooth mass of bone arising from the cortex with active periosteal rersponseOsteogenic sarcoma: proliferating bony lesions with the evidence of bone invasion and active new bone proliferation at its margins and sclerosis: "Sun Burst" Appearance |
| Bony cyst | Characterized by well demarcated radiolucent area within the bone and may be associated with cortical thinning or from bone expansion. |

*Contd.*

| **Radiological pathology of spinal cord** | |
|---|---|
| Spondylosis | Reduced intervertebral space |
| | Lipping of newborn from the ventral border between the two vertebrae |
| | In later stages, complete bridging of bony callus between the ventral vertebral surfaces |
| Intervertebral disc protrusion | Narrowing, wedging or collapse of the disc spaces |
| | Mineralized disc mass may be present within the epidural space to form radioopaque mechanical obstruction |
| | In myelographic examination, deviation of spinal cord is seen. |
| **Radiological pathology of thorax** | |
| Cardiomegaly | Outline of the heart becomes more rounded |
| | Occupies a much larger area of the thorax |
| | Trachea and major blood vessels are seen displaced |
| | Posterior border of heart become straighter |
| | Cardiac silhouette in contact with sternum and diaphragm |
| Dirofilariasis | Pulmonary artery shows increased prominence |
| | Right heart enlagement |
| | Consolidation (fluid filled) of lungs, in advance stage |
| Pericardial effusion | A very large and round heart shadow coupled with no stasis in the lungs, only a slight increase in density |
| Bronchitis | Slight increase in the radio-density of the bronchial tree |
| Pneumonia | Areas of increased density in lung substance consolidation (fluid filled) of the parenchyma |
| Pneumothorax | Collapse of the lungs leaving an "empty space" in the thoracic cavity |
| | Presence of air in the pleural cavity |
| | Floating heart shadow |
| Fluid in the pleural cavity | Diffuse radiographic density of both lungs |
| | Fluid level appears as area of increased density |
| | Typical leafy appearance |
| Diaphragmatic hernia | Disappearance of the normal diaphragm line/ contour of the diaphragm lost |
| | Heart may be displaced cranially |
| | Large irregular densities in the thoracic cavity |

*Contd.*

| | |
|---|---|
| Tuberculosis | Areas of opacity in lung parenchymacalcified and fibrotic nodules in the lung parenchyma or pleurapoorly defined pulmonary vessels |
| **Radiological pathology of abdomen** | |
| Gastric torsion | Marked distended and gas filled stomach |
| | Occupying the major portion of the anterior abdomen |
| | Compartalisation of the stomach |
| Esophageal achalasia | Distended organ occupying the upper half of the chest in the lateral view |
| | Dorso-ventral view-distended organ projectile beyond the shadow of the spine |
| Esophageal foreign body | Thickening of the oesophageal wall increased density from that of the surrounding tissues |
| Pyloric obstruction | Enlargement of the stomach |
| | Accumulation of the fluid/ material (accumulation of barium) in the pyloric area |
| Intussusception | Contrast agents would not pass beyond intussusceptions when barium enema is given. |
| | Barium enema-"coiled watch spring" pattern |
| | Sausage shaped mass with increased density |
| | Thin layer of gas outlining the layers of intussusceptions |
| Impacted ileum | Presence of dense masses and gas in the bowel |
| Obstructive ileums | The "gathered-flounce" pattern is pathgnomonic for obstructions caused by a piece of string or object |
| Perforated bowel | Increased density with diffuse contours of the abdominal organs |
| Hydronephrosis | Large mass with a smooth outline in the anterior abdomen filled with fluids, with appreence of homogenous density |
| Kidney calculi | Radioopaque calculi can be seen in the sublumbar renal area by intravenous pyelography |
| Ureteral calculi | Radioopaque structure in the mid abdomen |
| | Intravenous pyelogram would reveal enlarged kidney and dilatation on the affected side |
| Rupture of the gall bladder | Distended abdomen with ground glass appearance |
| | Increased density of the abdominal organs |
| Ruptured urinary bladder | Loss of bladder outline or bladder size markedly reduced |

*Contd.*

| | |
|---|---|
| | On retrograde urocystogram, the contrast agent would leak into the abdominal cavity |
| Splenomegaly | Presence of an elongated mass When spleen is invaded by tumour, the density of the enlarged spleen would be uneven |
| Prostate enlargement | Enlarged mass in the area of urinary bladder |
| | The urinary bladder may be displaced and obstacle to the passage through the rectum may be observed. |
| Paraprostatic cysts | Large soft tissue mass in caudal abdomen |
| | Contrast studies often required to identify the bladder from the cyst and vice versa. |
| | May lie dorsal, lateral to the bladder which is displaced accordingly. |
| Ovarian mass | Soft tissue mass located in mid abdomen-often more dorsally located than splenic masses. |
| | Ovarian neoplasia is most commonly unilateral but can be bilateral. |
| Uterine enlargement | Increased gap between bladder and descending colon. Multiple homogenous fluid filled loops of uterine horn seen in mid and caudal abdomen. |
| Pyometra and metritis | Slight thickening and enlagement of uterus-may be uniformly tubular or sacculated |
| | Gas filled distended uterine loop |
| | Displacement of the colon |
| Emphysematous fetuses | Uterus full of emphysematous disintegrating fetuses |
| | Under inflammatory conditions, gas filled fluid uterus may be observed. |

## Chapter - 20

# Contrast Agents and Special Radiography

**Contrast radiography:** The radiographic technique which employ the use of contrast media to identify a soft tissue structure or an organ and pathological findings which may be difficult or even impossible to visualize clearly in plain films due to lack of contrast with surrounding tissue is known as contrast radiography. This is a special radiographic techniques/procedures may be required to supplement or confirm the information obtained from plain or survey radiography.

The substances used for this purpose is called contrast agents/ medium/materials.

### Advantages

- The structure or organ can be more effectively evaluated for its size, shape and position.
- Used to gain information about the mucosal surface of a viscera or its luminal content.
- To evaluate organ functions.

### Principle and Type of Contrast Agent

- The substances used for this purpose are usually of high atomic number (Z, above 50) *e.g.* compounds of Barium (56) or Iodine (53) are radio opaque to X-rays. Since these substances increases radio density of the structure or tissue in relation to surrounding tissue (positive contrast to soft tissues) are called positive contrast agent.

- Gases (air or oxygen) which have low specific gravity are more radio lucent to X-rays than soft tissue. Since these are relatively decreases the radio density are called negative contrast agent.
- When both positive and negative contrast agents are used together to visualized a particular organ, it is called as double contrast study (*e.g.* Urinary bladder or alimentary tract). Occasionally it is accompanied by pneumoperitoneum for better visualization of serosal layer to.
- They may be injected into blood vessels either for the immediate visualization of vascular supply *e.g.* Arteriography or for their subsequent excretion through an organ *e.g.* kidney, liver.

**Classification radiographic contrast agents:**

| Generic name | Trade name | Uses | Dose |
|---|---|---|---|
| A).Positive contrast agents | Contain high atomic number that attenuate X-rays with great efficiency, increasing their radiographic opacity. | | |
| 1.Barium sulphate preparation (Powder, paste and suspension form) | Powder: Micropaque, Microtrast, Baritop-G Paste: Microtrast Suspension: Micropaqe, Baritop-100, Microbar. | Alimentary tract | 5-10 ml/kg body weight (25%)10-20 ml/kg body weight (20%)-enema |
| 2.Water soluble iodine compounds | Opaque to X-rays very soluble in water, low viscosity, low toxicity and low irritancy. | | |
| a).Ionic preparation (iodine content, mg/ml) | Are monomeric or dimeric derivatives of benzoic acid containing iodine that have a high atomic number and appear opaque (white) on radiograph. | | |
| Meglumine diatrizoate (390) | Hypaque 65% | Alimentary tract | 0.5 ml/kg body weight oral |
| Sodium diatrizoate (440) | Gastrografin | | |
| Sodium iothalamate (420) | Gastroconray | | |
| Sodium diatrizoate (440) | Hypaque | Urography, cystography, | 850 mg/kg body weight |

*Contd.*

| | | | |
|---|---|---|---|
| | | angiography, urethrography, hysterography, osteomedullo -graphy | intravenously |
| Meglumine iothalamate (280) | Conray | | |
| Meglumine /sodium diatrizoate | Renografin, Urografin | | |
| b).Non-ionic preparation (iodine content, mg/ml) | Are monomeric (most common) and dimeric derivatives of benzoic acid. Generally lower osmolality than ionic compounds. Excreated almost exclusively by the kidneys and relatively expansive. | | |
| Metrizamide (300) | Amipaque | Myelography, angiography, intravenous pyelography, Antrhography | 0.22 ml/kg body weight |
| Iohexol (140, 180, 300,350) | Omniaque | | |
| Iopamidol (200,300,370) | Niapam | | |
| 3.Viscous and oily agents | These agents are less irritant.<br>Because of their immiscibility with water, these preparations are not suitable for intravascular use.<br>Since water soluble contrast agents are quickly eliminated, viscous and oily preparations are indicated when this is not desirable character. | | |
| Iophendylate (300) | Myodil | Sialography | |
| Propylidone (280) | Dinosil | Bronchography | |
| Iodised seed oil (480) | Lipiodol | Dacrocystor -hinography, lymphangio -graphy | |
| 4.Cholycystopaques (Preparation excreted through biliary system) | These agents are largely excreted by liver and outline gall bladder and bile duct. These are water soluble organic iodine preparation. | | |
| Meglumine ioglycamate | Biligram | Cholecystography | intravenous |
| Iopanoic acid | Telepaque | Cholecystography | oral |
| Meglumine iodoxamate | Endobil | Cholecystography | |
| Meglumine iodipamide | Cholegrafin, Biligrafin | Cholecystography | |

*Contd.*

| | | | |
|---|---|---|---|
| B).Negative contrast agents: | Are gases with low physical density and low X-ray attenuation, therefore decreasing radiographic opacity. They are easily available,cheap and safe. It should be inert, quickly dissolved in the body fluid and quickly eliminated through the body. Used along with positive contrast agents for double contrast agent which gives best mucosal details and avoids complete oblitation of calculi or small foreign bodies. | | |
| Oxygen/air/ $Co_2$ | Pneumocystography<br>Arthography<br>Fasciagraphy<br>Pneumoperitoneography | | 4-10 ml/kg body weight |

## Prerequisite

- Contrast studies are not an excuse for poor quality radiography. Plain film must be taken prior to any contrast techniques.
- Adequate technical quality to avoid the necessity for repeat film during the contrast examination.
- A possible diagnosis that might obviate the need for a contrast study.
- To check that the patient has been adequately prepared for the contrast examination.
- To make sure that the contrast procedures chosen is the most appropriate to help with diagnosis.
- To help estimate the amount of contrast agent will be required for the procedure.

## Properties of an Ideal Contrast Agent

- The contrast agents or its metabolites should be non-toxic or non-carcinogenic.
- They should remain in the area of interest for desired duration.
- It should have desired atomic number (Z).
- It should be low viscosity and osmolarity.
- It should have high organ specificity.

## Adverse Reactions

- **Minor reactions:** Nausea, vomiting,urticaria

- **Intermediate reaction:** Bronchospasm, hypotension, persistence of minor reactions.
- **Major reactions:** Severe bronchospasm, severe hypotension, shock, convulsion, cardiac arrest.

**Different contrast radiographic techniques:**

| Techniques | Structure/Organ | Indications |
|---|---|---|
| Barium series | Alimentary tract | Obstruction by radiolucent foreign bodies, oesophageal defects (megaoesophageal dilatation), displacement of alimentary tract (hernia), lesions of lumen of GI tract (ulcers, neoplasm, growth) |
| Esophagography | Esophagous | |
| Reticulography | Reticulum | Reticular hernia |
| Barium enema | Colon and rectum | To visualization |
| Excretory urography | Kidney | Renal mass lesions, neoplasm, renal cyst, pyelonephritis, hydroureter, hydronephrosis, renal agesis, hypoplasia, pelvis urethral obstruction (calculi, clot), ectopic ureter. |
| Retrograde urethrography | Urethra | Strictures, trauma, lower urinary disorders like urethral crystalluria, proteinuria, calculi |
| Pneumocystography, positive cystography, double contrst cystography | Urinary bladder | |
| Myelography (injection of contrast agent into subarchnoid space) | Subarchnoid space of spinal cord | Spinal cord trauma, cord dislocation, disc herniation |
| Bronchography | Tracheal and bronchial structures | Bronchiectasis, bronchogenic, carcinoma, partial lung collapse and bronchoiostenosis |
| Cholecystography | Gall bladder | Gall stones |
| Pneumoperitoneo -graphy (introduction of air into the peritoneal cavity to outline the viscera) | Peritoneal cavity | Peritoneal adhesion, imperforated diaphragm, tumours of kidney, liver, pancrease, ovary, lymph gland |

| | | |
|---|---|---|
| Pleurography | Pleuropulmonary space | lesions |
| Arthrography (injection of contrast agent into the joint cavity) | Joint cavity | Chronic joint disease,osteo-arthritis, osteo chondrosis, joint mice, anlylosis |
| Angiography: Cardio angiography, cerebral angiography, renal angiography, spinal angiography (to study the vascular system following introduction of water soluble contrast agents in it) | Vascular system | Vascular occlusion, vascular pathology, aneurysm and vascular rupture |
| Lymphography | Lymph vessel and lymph nodes | Lymphatic abnormality and extent of lymph node involvement in metastasis |
| Siaolography | Salivary gland | Salivary calculi, salivary fistula |
| Dacrocystorhino -graphy(to study the patency of naso-lacrimal duct) | Naso-lacrimal duct | Patency of duct |
| Osteo medulography | Medullary cavity of bone | Fracture healing, bone grafting, diagnosis of bone disease |
| Fasciagraphy (technique to demonstrate adhesion around the tendons) | Tendon | Lameness, tenorryhaphy, tendon grafting, soft tissue healing around the joint |
| Fistulography (to determine the extend of origin of fistular tract) | Fistular tract | Evaluate fistulous tract |
| Sinus tract injection (contrast radiography is used in the investigation of sinus tracts, abscess cavities) | Sinus tract, abscess | Evaluate and explore sinus tract and abscess |
| Hysterosalpingo -graphy (technique is used to outline the uterus, fallopian tubes an ovary) | Uterus, fallopian tubes an ovary | Pyometra, metritis |

*Contd.*

| | | |
|---|---|---|
| Interosseous vertebral venography (positive contrast agents are injected into the body of the vertebra caudal to the suspected site of lesion. This opacity of the vertebral veins located at the floor of the vertebral canal) | Vertebral canal | Spinal concussion, spinal<br><br>Trauma |

## Examination of Alimentary Tract

### Indications

- Complete obstruction by non-radioopaque foreign bodies.
- Congenital abnormalities in esophagus, stomach and bowel.
- Abnormal displacement of alimentary tract due to the pressure of an intra-abdominal mass in association with ruptured diaphragm.
- Lesions on the wall of the alimenatary tract *e.g.* Neoplasm, ulcers *etc.*

Barium swallow (esophagography): dynamic (with fluoroscopy) or static (with radiography) contrast study of the pharynx and esophagus.

### Technique

Place the animal in lateral recumbency. Administer barium sulphate about 50 to 100 gms as a paste orally. For each administration of contrast agent, monitor swallowing and transport of contrast to the stomach with fluoroscopy or with lateral and ventro dorsal radiographs are made post swallowing.

### Barium meal (Stomach)

### Technique

50 to 100% suspension of about 15 to 100 ml is given orally observed under fluoroscopy or X –rays are taken at regular intervals of 10-20 minutes, 1 hour and 4 hrs *etc.* at different angles like lateral, right lateral, ventrodorsal and oblique to demonstrate the different

areas of stomach and mucosal surface. Stomach should be emptied before the procedure. Double contrast gastrography can be obtained by combining of air.

**Reticulography:** Barium suspensions (1-2 kg) is given orally and obtain lateral radiography after 40 minutes with the animal in lateral or supine position.

## Small Intestine

To promote easy passage of contrast agent 25% suspension is preferred. Repeated radiograph at different intervals will demonstrate lesions inside or outside the intestine easily.

## Large Intestine

To demonstrate the large intestine, barium is given as an anema. Double contrast colonography can be obtained by combing air.

## Urinary System

## Intravenous Pyelography/ Excretory Urography

Contrast procedure designed to enhance visualization of the kidneys, renal pelvis and ureters.

## Indications

- To assess shape, size and position of kidneys, ureters and bladder.
- To increase the definition of the kidney shadow when it cannot be identified in a survey radiograph
- To show the presence or absence of lesion of kidney pelvis (calculi)

## Preparation

- The animal is fasted for 12 – 24 hrs.
- Cleansing enema is given.
- Survey radiograph is taken.
- Patient is placed in dorsal recumbency.
- The contrast agent *e.g.* iohexol is infused intravenously @ 3ml/kg body weight in dogs.

- The animal is turned to ventrodorsal position.
- Exposure of the animal is done immediately to get nephrogram phase of kidney.
- Lateral and ventrodorsal radiographs are taken @ 5,10,20,30 minutes to get pyelogram, uterogram, cystogram are obtained.
- Use of compression bandage over the abdomen will enhance the clarity of renal pelvis and ureter.

**Cystography:** It is the technique of introducing the contrast agents into the urinary bladder through a catheter.

## Indications

- To aid in the recognition of small cystic calculi or those of low radio-opacity.
- To demonstrate neoplasia or other lesions of the wall of the urinary bladder such as mural lesions, rupture of the bladder.
- To assist in radiography of prostatic conditions by demonstrating displacement of the urinary bladder by an abnormal prostate gland.
- To correlate in animals unresponsive conditions such as haematuria, crystluria, bacteria, dysuria, anuria and urinary incontinence.

## Technique

- Animal is sedated.
- 3 to 5 french sterile polypropylene red rubber catheter is introduced through urethra using lignocaine get.
- All the urine present in the bladder is aspirated by means of a syringe.
- Blood clots if present in the bladder is flushed out with the help of a syringe.
- Contrast agent iohexol @ 10 ml/kg is introduced mixed with normal saline.
- The bladder is palpated in the abdomen if found distended the infusion is stopped.

- Lateral and vendrodorsal radiographs are taken. For male dogs oblique view is preferred.

**Urethrography:** Contrast study designed to enhance visualization of the urethra. It is the contrast technique of filling the urethra with contrast agents (water soluble iodinated or air , carbon dioxide) to detect urethral trauma, stricture, obstruction, tumour *etc.*

## Technique

- The animal is sedated.
- Balloon tip catheter is introduced into the urethra and inflated.
- Tip of the catheter is at the tip of urethra.

*Patient preparation:* Fast 12-24 hours and use of cleansing enema (administer 4 hrs before study to minimize gas artifact).

## Retrograde Urethrogram

- Fill the lumen of the catheter with contrast agent before placement into the urethra.
- Insert the lubricated tip ot the catheter 1 -3 cm into the urethral orifice and inflate the ballon.
- Inject 3-20 ml of contrast agent into the urethra.
- Make the exposure during infusion, toward the end of the injection.
- Repeat the injection for ventrodorsal and oblique projections, if necessary.

## Antegrade (voiding) Urethrogram

- With the bladder distended with a positive contrast agent, place gentle pressure on the bladder with a paddle or wooden spoon.
- Exposure is taken when urine is noted at the uretheral orifice.

## Spinal Cord

## Myelography

Myelography is an X-ray examination of the spinal canal. A contrast agent is injected through a needle into the subarachnoid space to display the spinal cord, spinal canal, and nerve roots on an X-ray.

When the contrast agent is injected into the subarachnoid space, the radiologist is able to view and evaluate the status of the spinal cord, the nerve roots and the meninges. It may be done in the neck area (cisternal myelogram,) or in the lower back area(lumbar myelogram).

## Indications of Myelography

Myelography is most commonly used to detect abnormalities affecting the spinal cord, the spinal canal, the spinal nerve roots and the blood vessels that supply the spinal cord.

It is indicated when focal spinal cord lesion is suspected and no inflammatory response is seen on cerebrospinal fluid (CSF) analysis.

The contrast agents mix with CSF that surrounds the spinal cord and demonstrates focal spinal cord compression or expansion. Myelography is performed in following conditions:

- Where the neurological examination indicates a particular spinal lesion, but none is visible on plain radiography.
- To show whether a herniation of the intervertebral disk between the successive vertebral bodies is compressing the nerve roots or the spinal cord,
- To depict a condition that often accompanies degeneration of the bones and soft tissues surrounding the spinal canal, termed spinal stenosis. In this condition, the spinal canal narrows as the surrounding tissues enlarge due to the development of bony spurs (osteophytes) and thickening of the adjacent ligaments.
- It can also be used to assess the following conditions when MR imaging cannot be performed, or in addition to MRI (when MR does not provide sufficient information): tumors involving the bony spine, meninges, nerve roots or spinal cord; infection involving the bony spine, intervertebral discs, meninges and surrounding soft tissues; inflammation of the arachnoid membrane that covers the spinal cord; spinal lesions caused by disease or trauma.
- Patients with known cancer who develop back pain may require a myelogram for evaluation.
- To assist in deciding the indications for surgery and type of procedure to be performed.

## Procedure of Myelography

The contrast agent usually is injected into the lower lumbar spinal canal, because it is considered easier and safer. Occasionally, if it is deemed safer or more useful, the contrast agent will be injected into the upper cervical spine. At the site of the injection, the skin will be cleaned and then numbed with a local anesthetic. Depending on the location of the puncture, the patient will be positioned. The needle is advanced, usually under fluoroscopic guidance, until its tip is positioned within the subarachnoid space within the spinal canal, at which time a free slow flow of fluid is obtained. If requested by the referring physician, a small amount of cerebrospinal fluid may be withdrawn and sent for laboratory studies. The contrast agent is then injected through the needle, the needle is removed and the skin at the puncture site is again cleaned. The patient is then positioned on the table, usually lying on their ventral side. Under fluoroscopic guidance, the radiologist then slowly tilts the X-ray table allowing the contrast agent to flow up or down within the subarachnoid space and to surround the nerve roots or the spinal cord. As the table is tilted, the radiologist monitors the flow of contrast material with fluoroscopy, focusing on the area that correlates with the patient's symptoms. At this point, the patient may be repositioned on his/her side, and additional X-ray images may be obtained by the radiologist, while such images are being obtained, it is important for the patient to remain still to reduce the possibility of blurred images. When these images have been completed, the table is returned to the horizontal position, and the patient is allowed to roll onto his/her back and assume a position of greater comfort while the images are checked by the radiologist. A computed tomography (CT) scan is frequently performed immediately following the conclusion of the myelography while contrast agent is still present within the spinal canal to better define the anatomy and any abnormalities. This combination of imaging studies is known as CT myelography. A myelography examination is usually completed within 30 to 60 minutes. A CT scan will add another 15 to 30 minutes to the total examination time. In most cases, the myelogram is followed by a computed tomography (CT) scan Magnetic resonance imaging (MRI) is often the first imaging exam done to evaluate the spinal cord and nerve roots. However, on occasion, a patient has a medical device, such as a cardiac pacemaker and with spinal instrumentation (screws, plates, rods, etc.). MRI may not be optimal because of artifacts generated by these instruments that may prevent from undergoing MRI. In such cases, myelography and/or a CT scan, in lieu of MRI, is performed to better define abnormalities.

## Contrast Agents

The selection of contrast agents has a crucial role in myelographic examination. The ideal contrast preparation, should be minimal neurotoxic, should be pharmacologically inert, miscible with CSF and radio opaque at an isotonic concentration. A number of contrast media have been recommended for myelography, which include ionic and non-ionic monomers of benzoic acid. Various contrast agents are:

1. **Non-ionic water-soluble contrast agents:** Nonionic contrast must be used for the examination. Intrathecal administration of Ionic iodinated contrast can cause death. They are Metrizamide, Omnipaque (Iohexol) and Iopamidol (Isovue). Omnipaque (Iohexol) comes in 20-ml vials with concentrations of 180 mg I/ml and 300 mg I/ml. Recommended volumes of contrast agents for myelography in dogs are generally accepted to be 0.3-0.4 ml/kg. Before drawing the contrast into the syringe, the technologist should show you the bottle. Verify that the expiration date has not passed and the desired concentration of contrast (180 or 300 mg I/ml) is being used.
2. **Oil based contrast agents:** They are Pentoplaque, Thorotrast, Neo-ipex (75%), Idochlorol, Skiodon (20%), Lipidal and Diodrast (35%) are various type media. Vaughan, 1990 listed various disadvantages of oil-based contrast medium such as poor diagnostic quality, poor flow characteristics, tendency to globulate, and post myelographic arachnoiditis. Because of the above disadvantages oil based contrast media are no longer used.

## Technique of Myelography

I) **Cisternal Myelography:** An angle of 45-60$^{o}$ tilt with head held high at highest position for 3-5 minutes.

## Advantages

- Provides easy access to sub-arachnoid space allowing collection of requisite amount of CSF with minimum chances of blood contamination. Needle insertion is technically easier.
- Less contrast agent is required for evaluation of cervical lesions.

## Disadvantages

- Sub-dural injection is most common complication observed during cisternal injection of contrast agent.
- Post-procedural seizures.
- Slight risk of needle puncture into medulla oblongata or cervical spinal cord.

II) **Lumbar Myelography:** General anaesthesia is administered to the patient. The back is arched dorsally with patient in sternal recumbancy. A 3-inch 22 G needle with syringe is introduced in the midline just anterior to L6 space. Cerebrospinal fluid 1-3 ml is removed for examination and agent is injected slowly and carefully. The spine should be tilted for some time toward the head (20°) to encourage cranial migration. Radiographs are made on similar intervals as cisterna magna myelography.

## Advantages

- It is safer than cisternal puncture.
- It is useful for compressive lesions of thoracolumbar region.
- More useful in cases with acute disc prolapse.

## Disadvantages

- Technically it is more difficult than cisternal myelography .
- Various side effects of lumbar myelography as spinal cord edema, cystic necrosis, myelomalacia, axonal necrosis and hydromelia.

III). **Lumbosacral Myelography:** tilt of 60° anterior-posteriorly and found dye satisfactorily traveled to lumbosacral region within 5 min.

## Advantages

- Spinal cord terminates at caudal lumbar so there is minimal risk for cord injury.
- Lumbosacral myelography is less difficult because of large space.
- Puncture site is easily palpable

## Disadvantages

- Seizures are observed after myelography.

## Difficulties in Myelography

- *Poor radiographic quality:* incorrect patient positioning, incorrect exposure or artifact results into poor radiographic quality. Myelography should be performed only after satisfactory quality survey radiographs have been obtained and carefully examined.
- *Poor distribution of contrast agents :* inadequate volume injected; incorrect injection site; epidural opacification; contrast not inadequately mixed with CSF; incorrect radiographic views
- *Patho-anatomical problems:* normal anatomical variations; spinal cord swelling.

## Evaluation

The contrast study should be evaluated for the following features:

- Demonstration of complete or partial obstruction to the flow of contrast columns outlining the subarchnoid space.
- Evidence of complete or partial obstruction to the flow of contrast.
- Displacement of deviation of the contrast columns.
- Variation in width of the contrast columns or filling defects.
- Outlining by the contrast columns of extra dural masses.
- Divergence of the contrast columns indicative of intr-medullary lesions, cord swelling or cord compression in the other place.

# Chapter - 21

# Radiography of Exotic Animals and Birds

Radiology has been an important diagnostic modality in exotic animals and birds (includes rodents, reptiles and fish). The radiographic equipment needed for radiography of exotic animals and birds is basically the same to that used for domestic animals. A high-milliamperage (mA) X-ray machine, having 200- or 300 mA unit is recommended to allow the use of a short exposure time (1/40 seconds) or less are preferred. Maximum kilovoltage (kVp, 40-75) is less important for avian and exotic radiography than for domestic animal radiography. As with other species, at least two radiographic views at $90^0$ angles to each other are recommended. However, restraining and knowledge of radiographic anatomy of different species of exotic animals and birds are the prerequisite for the modality. Restrain and immobilization:

Physical restraint like plexiglass sheet/tubes, ropes, sandbags and other devices (radilucent sheet/plastic sheet) may be used for radiographic study.

- **Chemical immobilization**

  Ketamine hydrochloride and phencyclidine derivates have been greatly facilitated the positioning of the animals. By using these drugs, it is possible to position the patients properly for radiographic examination to minimize stress and trauma to the patient and to avoid hazard as physical restraining by the personnel is not required.

- **Radiographic anatomy**

  Normal radiographic reference of various species of exotic animals and birds of different ages and sexes is to be developed. This will help to recognize any abnormality.]

## Radiographic Positioning

- **Reptiles**

  **Turtles and tortoise**

  Whole body: cranio-caudal view, lateral view (horizontal beam), dorsoventral view (vertical beam).

  - *Lizard:* DV (vertical beam), lateral view (horizontal beam).
  - *Snakes and rodent:* DV (vertical beam), lateral view (horizontal beam).

- **Nonhuman primates**

  *Thorax:* VD and lateral erect view.

  *Abdomen:* VD and lateral recumbent view.

- *Birds:*

  Whole body survey- lateral views; wings and leg: lateral and caudocranial view.

- *Fish:*

  A dorsoventral view of a fish can be obtained by placing in a sealable plastic bag with enough water to allow respiration.

  An alternate method of obtaining a lateral view requires rapid preparation and exposure by the radiographer.

## Chapter - 22

# Advance Diagnostic Imaging Tools and Techniques

Diagnostic imaging refers to technologies that doctors use to look inside the body of the patient for clues about any disease condition. A variety of machine and techniques can create pictures of the structures and activities inside the patient body. In India, some of these modalities like digital radiography and ultrasonography are being used at some of the veterinary colleges and reaseach institutes while at some places some of the veterinarians have access to the techniques like computed tomography (CT) and magnetic resoncace imaging (MRI) of the human hospitals. So this is the responsibility of the scientists and researchers engaged in the advancement of the diagnostic imaging and the manufacturing companies to make these facilities cot effective so that an animal of a common man can be benefited with these facilities.

Diagnosis refers to the process of attempting to determine a possible disease or ailments. A clinician uses several sources of data and puts the pieces of related information together to make a diagnostic impression. After the initial diagnostic impression, clinician obtain follow up procedures and tests to get more data to support or reject the original diagnosis and will attempt to narrow it down to a more specific level. Diagnostic procedures are the specific tools that the clinicians use to narrow the diagnostic possibilities. The plural of diagnosis is *diagnoses,* the verb is to *diagnose,* and a person who diagnoses is called a *diagnostician.*

## Significance of Diagnostic Imaging

It enables visual evaluation of normal and abnormal anatomy.

- It enhances the clinicians level of diagnostic accuracy.
- Endow with method of closely monitor therapy.

**Various diagnostic imaging procedures can be classified as follows:**

1. *Anatomic imaging:* Radiology, Fluoroscopy, Image Intensifier, Rapid serial radiography, Digital radiography, Direct digital radiography, Computed radiography, Positron emission tomography, Xeroradiography, Subtraction technique, Ultrasonography, Magnetic resonance imaging, Magnetic resonance spectroscopy, Functional Magnetic resonance imaging.
2. *Physiologic imaging:* Nuclear scientigraphy, Scientigraphy positron emission tomography or single photon emission computed tomography, Diagnostic thermogrphy
3. *Scope:* Endoscope/Laparoscope
4. Interventional imaging

**Radiology:** Conventional radiography is usually the initial method continues to be mainstay of diagnostic imaging in third world countries. Radiograph is a two-dimensional depiction of a three-dimensional object.

## Flouroscopy

- Continuous viewing of the image as X-rays pass through the patient is flouroscopy.
- Sometimes incorrectly termed screening is the dynamic radiological study of the body parts.
- Fluoroscope is a device used to view an X-ray image on a fluorescent screen instead of the film. The X-rays after passing through the body parts are transformed into visible light which is observed on a screen coated with filament material, either directly or through an intensifying device.

## Advantages

Simple, save time and expenses of exposing and developing a film, provide dynamic radiographic study.

## Disadvantages

More radiation hazard. Accommodation in dark vision is necessary. Smaller details are escaped as intensity of image is low.

## Uses of Fluoroscopy

1) Clinical examination of the dynamics of the body such as peristalsis and movement of joints.
2) Proper placement of catheter in bronchus during broncography.
3) Study of birth postures of fetus.
4) Position of pins or nails during orthopedic surgery.

## Instrumentation

Is composed of a fluoroscopic screen suspended over the examination table with a fixed attachement to an X-ray tube under the table. The screen is coated with cadmium zinc sulfide crystals which emit green light. Many fluoroscopes are equipped with spot film to record the fluoroscopic image and image intensified fluoroscopy for better resolution.

## Image Intensifier

An image intensifier is an electronic unit that receives primary X-ray beam after passing through the patient's body and allows it to fall on the input phosphor (layer of fluorescent material) of the image intensifier tube. Image intensification through an image intensifier overcomes problems to large extent, which were encountered with fluoroscopy like lack of brightness and increased radiation hazard. The provision of recoding motion of an organ is known as cinefluorography.

## Advantages

- The image produced for viewing is 1000-5000 times brighter than that obtained by conventional fluoroscopic unit.
- Brightness and contrast of the image can be electronically controlled
- It is possible to record the motion of organs through a recording system.

- Spot film camera can be used.
- Lower mA settings- low radiation hazard.
- Image can be viewed on TV.

## Disadvantage

Expensive

## Rapid Serial Radiography

Multiple serial exposures on large conventional size X-ray film. Two basic types of equipment are available, one that moves a loaded cassette and other that moves only radiographic film in a cut or roll format.

## Digital Radiography

Digital images can be electronically stored, transmitted, processed and displayed under computer control. It is based on storage phosphor technology in an imaging system in which X-ray images are correctly exposed due to storage screens extremely wide exposure range. It offers virtually endless opportunities for qualititative and quantitative image assessment. Bone and soft tissues are clearly visible from a single exposure. It is possible that a day will come when x-ray films will no longer be used in radiography.

## Direct Digital Radiography

Special digital panel (solid state detector) with cable directly to computer (some are wireless). Here no reader step is needed-X-ray direct to digital panel and digital panel reused. Radiograph produced one is a digital image.

## Advantages of Digital Radiography (either CR or DR):

- No wet processing required; better consistency of X-rays.
- No darkroom required -saves space; no consumables.
- Chemistry–reduces costs and protects environment.
- No rooms full of filing cabinets of X-ray images; reduction of artifacts: improves image quality.
- Higher quality images and thus more accurate diagnosis. It should be noted that digital radiography will not improve image quality where bad radiographic technique is used.

- Manipulation of image to highlight different detail (bone or soft tissue) or compensate for exposure: reduces the number of re-takes and exposures.
- Share images via email or CD and thus quicker referral.
- Multiple plates of varying sizes, similar to existing cassette/ screen: maintains existing flexibility image capture time substantially reduced from wet processing and thus saves time.

## Disadvantage of Digital Radiography (either CR or DR)

- Do not have the degree of spatial resolution possible with film-screen radiography. However, this is of little clinical relevance and is overcome by its advantages.
- This may increase the cost in purchasing the computer in the examination room.

## Computed Radiography

Imaging plate (instead of film) traps X-rays energy on photostimulable phosphor as latent image. Imaging plate put into a reader. Scanning laser beam caused light to be released which is then converted into electrical signal for image. Images plate is cleared and reused. This type of radiograph is a digital image.

## Xeroradiography

It is the method of X-ray imaging in which visible electrostatic charged pattern is produced on the surface of photoconductor. Amorphous selenium is used as a photoconductor on a xeroradiographic plate. Thus a latent image is formed on the selenium coat of the plate by changing the electrostatic charges as per intensity of X-rays reaching the plates. This plate in now processed by exposing to and aerosol of charged power (toner). The toner particles are attracted or repelled by the electrostatic charge on the plate and thus an image is formed. This image is now transferred to plastic coated paper by direct contact and fused to the paper by heat.

**Applications:** In soft tissue imaging e.g., in radiographic examination of the mammary glands, muscles, tendons and ligaments.

## Advantage of Xeroradiography over Conventional Radiography

Include enhanced visualization of the borders between images of different densities (edge effect), good resolution, low contrast and wider exposure latitue which enables differentiation between fat, muscles and bones. The radiation exposure in xeroradiographs of the extremities less than that for nonscreen film radiography.

## Disadvantage

This technique cannot be used for very thick parts a very high exposure is required.

## Substraction Technique

It is a photographic technique that eliminates unwanted images from the radiograph and makes it easier to visualize important radiographic information on the radiograph. Principle is [A] and [B] radiographs are similar except [B] has additional information. To identify these letters a negative (C) of [A] is made. When (C) is superimposed on [B], order to clearly visualize the pattern and changes in vascular supply. For example in a cerebral angiogram the overlying bony structures make it difficult to critically examine the minute blood vessels. Now if these bones are somehow removed from the radiograph, even minute vessels will be clear. Therefore, to destroy the bony density we will require survey radiograph of the skull, an angiogram exactly in the same plane and without motion and a negative of the survey radiograph (called substraction mask). The bones will appear white on the survey radiograph and the angiogram, but opposite will be the case in the subtraction mask.

## Computed Axial Tomography (CAT /CT Scan)

CT is a diagnostic modality that is fundamentally different X-ray technique in which an organ is scanned in successive layers (cross sectional or transverse) by a narrow beam of X-rays, in such a way that the transmission of X-ray photons across a particular layer can be measured and by means of a computer, used to construct a picture of the internal structures.

## Principle

CT is based on the same basic principles of all other radiographic techniques, rays are absorbed or attenuated by materials in their path. As X-rays pass through the target organ they are absorbed in different tissues of the organs, the process is called attenuation. The degree of attenuation is related to the density and chemical structure of the organ. The attenuation is measured and stored in the memory of the computer. By computing this different attenuation co-efficient an image is displaced on the monitor. The resultant image is clearer than conventional radiography. The aim of the system is to produce a series of images by a tomographic method. The unique three dimensional anatomical visualization, non-invasive nature, ability to perform or quantitative tissue characterization is definitely a great hope for future of veterinary profession.

## Application

CT shall be able to provide a fairly good amount of diagnostic precision for various animal diseases.

## Positron Emission Tomography (PET)

PET is a nuclear medicine imaging technique which produces a three dimensional image or picture of functional processes in the body. The systems detect pairs of gamma rays emitted indirectly by a positron-emitting radionuclide (tracer), which is introduced into the bodt on a biologically active molecule. Images of tracer concentration in 3D or 4D space within the body are then reconstructed by computer analysis. Radioisotope emits positron-combine with electron-to form postronium-emits gamma rays-detected by crystal detectors-computer analysis-image are formed. It is a new area of metabolic imaging technique of future with exciting potential. When using PET, it is as if we are viewing th body with a microscope and pair of binoculars at the same time, that is looking at the cell and whole body at the same time.

Uses: brain tumor, epilepsy, central nervous system disorders and whole body can be imaged.

## Ultrasonographic Imaging Technique

It is the technique of visualizing the internal organs of the body (animal or human) using ultrasound waves. Ultrasound is characterized by sound waves with a frequency higher than the upper range of human hearing, approximately 20,000 cycles per second (20 kHz). 1 million cycles per second is 1 megahertz (MHz). Sound frequencies in the range of 2 to 10 MHz to create images of body structures based on the pattern of echoes reflected from the tissues and organs are commonly used in diagnostic examinations. A lot of advancements have been added to ultrasound imaging technology in recent years. Duplex and colour Doppler ultrasound, multihertz high-resolution tranducer, 3- dimensional ultrasound, 4-dimensional ultrasound, sonoendoscopic probes, ultrasound guided biopsy options have made the examination more versatile. Contrast enhanced ultrasonography with micro bubble contrast agent and tissue harmonic imaging (THI) are found very efficacious to study organ functioning and hemodynamic parameters. Ultrasonography is a potential armament in the hands of expert clinicians for diagnosis of various diseases/conditions in the light of clinical signs, laboratory findings and other diagnostic modalities. However, the examination takes skill and training to perform and to interpret. It it essential to produce an image of diagnostic quality that will allow the sinologist to differentiate between artifacts and real image. The sinologist must have a thorough knowledge of the instrumentation of the ultrasound machine and sound understanding of the anatomical position of the organ.

## Principle

A sound wave travels in a pulse and when it is reflected back it becomes an echo. It is the pulse-echo principle, which is used for ultrasound imaging. A pulse is generated by one or more piezoelectric crystals in an ultrasound transducer. When these crystals are stimulated electrically it changes its shape and produces sound waves of particular frequencies. The sound waves travel into the body and hit a boundary between tissues (e.g. between fluid and soft tissue, soft tissue and bone). Some of the sound waves reflect back to the probe, while some travel on further until they reach another boundary and then reflect back to the probe. The reflected waves are detected by the probe and relayed to the machine. The machine calculates the distance from the probe to the tissue or organ (boundaries) using the speed of sound in tissue (1540 m/s) and the time of the each echo's return (usually on the order of millionths of a second). The machine displays the distances and intensities of the echoes on the screen, forming a two dimensional (2D) image. In modern scanning systems, the sound beam is swept through the body many times per second, producing a dynamic, and real time image those changes as the transducer is moved across the body. This real-time image is easier to interpret and allows the examiner to scan continuously until a satisfactory image is obtained.

## Interactions of Ultrasound with Matter

Ultrasound interactions are determined by the acoustic properties of matter. As ultrasound energy propagates through a medium, interactions that occur include:

**Absorption:** It occurs when the energy in the sound beam is absorbed by the tissues thereby converting it into heat. Absorption process forms the basis of therapeutic ultrasound.

**Reflection:** A portion of the ultrasound beam is reflected at tissue interface. The sound reflected back toward the source is called an echo and is used to generate the ultrasound image. The percentage of ultrasound intensity reflected depends in part on the angle of incidence of the beam. As the angle of incidence increases, reflected sound is less likely to reach the transducer.

**Refraction:** Refraction is the change in direction of an ultrasound beam when passing from one medium to another with a different acoustic velocity. Ultrasound machines assume straight line propagation, and refraction effects give rise to artifacts.

**Scattering:** It occurs when the beam encounters an interface that is irregular and smaller than the sound beam. The portion of the beam that interacts with this interface is scattered in all the directions. Two closely related phenomenon occur, refraction and diffraction of which refraction is a common cause of artifacts. Acoustic scattering arises from objects within a tissue that are about the size of the wavelength of the incident beam or smaller, and represent a rough or non-specular reflector surface. As frequency increases, the non-specular (diffuse scatter) interactions increase, resulting in an increased attenuation and loss of echo intensity. Scatter gives rise to the characteristic speckle patterns of various organs, and is important in contributing to the grayscale range in the image.

**Attenuation:** Ultrasound attenuation, the loss of energy with distance traveled, is caused chiefly by scattering and tissue absorption of the incident beam (dB). The intensity loss per unit distance (dB/cm) is the attenuation coefficient.

*Rule of thumb:* Attenuation in soft tissue is approx. 1 dB/cm/MHz. The attenuation coefficient is directly proportional to and increases with frequency. Attenuation is medium dependent.

**Acoustic Impedance(Z ):** Is equal to density of the material times speed of sound in the material in which ultrasound travels. The differences between acoustic impedance values at an interface determine the amount of energy reflected at the interface.

**Acoustic Shadowing of Sound Wave:** Total reflection of sound waves at interfaces of bone, calcification and gas-filled structures. No imaging of area distal to reflective interface and shadowing is displayed as a uniform black area distal to reflector. Incomplete shadowing may appear distal to stones and calculi.

**Ultrasound Machine:** Large and small portable ultrasound machine suitable for different species of animals and type of examination are available in the market. Basic components are central processing unit (CPU); transducer probe; transducer pulse controls, display; keyboard/cursor; disk storage; printers.

**Transducer (probe or scan head):** Is a device that converts one form of energy to another. In U/S imaging this means converting electric energy into sound wave and vice versa. The frequency emitted by a particular transducer depends on the characteristics of the special piezoelectric crystal contained within the transducer. Transducer selection comes with experience, but general guidelines may help the new sonographer to select an appropriate frequency. For routine two-dimensional and M-mode echocardiography, cat and small dogs (< 7 kg) and small body parts (thyroid, breast), are usually examined initially with a higher frequency 7.5 to 10 MHz transducer. A 5 MHz transducer is used for most dogs and thick body parts (abdomen), except some large dogs (>50 kg), which may requires a lower frequency 3.0-3.5 MHz transducer. For optimal Doppler imaging, it may be necessary to sacrifice 2D image resolution and to use a lower frequency transducer than one would generally use for 2D or M -mode examination in the same patient.

## Types of Transducers

**Phased array transducers:** A sector field of view is produced by firing multiple transducer elements (64 to 128 elements) in a precise sequence electronically. The beam can be steered in different directions and focussed at various levels, which allows the transducer to have a small size yet a wide field of view at deeper depths.

**Linear array transducers:** A linear array transducer has multiple crystals (256 to 512) elements arranged in a line within a bar-shaped scan head. The narrow beam is swept through a rectangular field firing the transducers crystals sequentially to produces the ultrasound beam. These transducers come in variety of sizes and frequencies. Small rectangular linear array transducers are commonly used for small parts (abdominal- extra thoracic) scanning and sonography of superficial structure (skin, mammary gland, joints and tendons) in small animals.

**Curvilinear array transducers**: Are linear arrays shapes into convex curves. They produce a sector image that has a wider field of view than that of linear arrays. These transducers also come in variety of sizes and frequencies suitable for many general purpose applications. Trapezoid convex (curved array is useful in abdominal ultrasonography and pregnancy diagnosis).

**Mechanical sector scanners:** The real scanner is named bacuase the beam shape and resulting screen image produced by the transducer are triangular or pie shaped or sector shaped or fan shaped. A mechanical real-time sector scanner sweeps the beam through the field of view by movement of either solitary crystals or multiple crystals to generate real-time image. Mechanical sector scanners are less commonly used today because of the increased affordability of the various types of array scanners.

Sector scanners, whether mechanical or electronic, have the disadvantage of limited near field visibility compared with linear array or curvilinear array transducers. Sector scanners are particularly useful in echocardiography, sonography of intra pelvic and intra thoracic organs, brain, eyes, testes and joints.

## Modes of Echo Display

There are three modes of echo display which are used frequently in clinical applications in veterinary medicine.

**A-mode (amplitude mode):** Is the least frequently used. Used for ophthalmic examinations and other applications requiring precise length and depth measurements are needed.

**B-mode (brightness mode):** Displays the returning echoes as dots whose brightness or gray scale is proportional to the amplitude of the returned echo and whose position corresponds to the depth at which the echo originated along a single line (representing the beam's axis) from the transdrucer. B-mode is usually displayed with the transducer positioned at the top of the screen and depth increasing to the bottom of the screen. Used most often in clinical practice and produces 2 dimensional reconstruction of the image slice.

**M/TM- mode (Motion or Time-Motion mode):** Is used for echocardiography along with B-mode to evaluate the heart. M-mode tracing usually record depth on the vertical axis and time on the horizontal axis. The image is oriented with the transducer at the top. The motion of the dots (changes in distance of reflecting interfaces from the transducer) is recorded with respect to time. The echo tracings produced with M-mode are useful for precise cardiac chamber and wall measurements and quantitative evaluation of mitral valve leaflets or wall motion with time.

**Real time B-mode:** Displays a moving gray scale image of cross sectional anatomy. This is accomplished by sweeping a thin, focussed ultrasound beam across a triangular, linear or curvilinear field of view in the patient many times per second. The field is made up of many single B-mode lines. Sound pulses are sent out and echoes received back sequentially along each B-mode line of the field until a complete sector image is formed.

## Echogenicity

*Anechoic (echo free):* Tissues without acoustic interfaces appear as black area (fine or coarse).

*Hypoechoic (echo poor):* Tissues with low echogenicity appear medium to dark grey.Tissues with medium echogenicity appear light to medium grey.

*Hyperechoic (echo rich):* Echo rich tissues, calcification and gas filled organs appear as white or light grey.

**Image interpretation:** The proportion of sound waves reflected in represented on the ultrasound image by shades of gray ranging from black to white. The density of the tissue determines the shade of gray visualized on the screen. Gas and bone are barrier to ultrasound beam and appear white (hyperechoic) on the screen; ultrasound passes uninterrupted through fluid and appears black (anechoic) on screen; images of the soft tissues appear as shades of gray (hypoechoic) depending upon their proportion of fat, fibrous tissue and fluid. Following order of decreasing echogenicity of body tissues and substances.

Bone, gas, organ boundaries (more echogenic)> structural fat, vessel walls>renal sinus>prostate> spleen> storage fat>liver>renal cortex>muscle>renal medulla>bile, urine (least echogenic).

Doppler works on Doppler principle to the processing of reflected ultrasound waves. The principal value of these studies is the delineation of the direction and velocity of blood flow in the heart and great vessels.

**Artifacts in ultrasound:** Any density or mark on a ultrasound scan that is caused by something not belonging to the part of being imaged.

**Artifacts can be divided into two categories:**

Useless artifacts are produced by improper use of equipment, improper machine setting, improper scanning procedures or improper patient preparation. These artifacts usually affect the quality of images and therefore the interpretation.

Useful artifacts enhance accurate interpretation and are produced under proper technical conditions. The useful artifacts are a result of interactions ultrasound and matter.

## Artifact Production

**Reverberation:** Refers to the production of spurious echoes due to two or more reflectors in the sound path; the first reflector is usually the skin-transducer interface (external reverberation). Internal reflector such as bone or gas is also common causes of reverberation (internal reverberation). For example: gas filled bowel segments. The sound is entirely reflected back from the gas and then bounces back and forth between probe and the gas creating multiple echoes from one ultrasound transducer.

**Mirror-image artifacts:** Are produces by rounded, strongly reflective interfaces such as the diaphragm-lung interface. Part of the insonating beam is reflected back into the liver. The echoes from the liver return to the transducer along the same path via the diaphragm-lung interface. The ultrasound machine assumes that the sound pulse and the reflected echoes travel to and from the transducer in a straight line. A mirror image is produced in this erroneous position because of the increased round- trip time.

**Side-lobe artifacts:** Lateral displacement of the structures not aligned with the sound beam is called side-lobe artifact. It is produced by minor beams of sound travelling out in directions different from the primary ultrasound beam. When side lobes of sufficient intensity interact with a highly reflective interface, the returning echoes are erroneously displaced along the path of the main ultrasound beam even though they did not originate within the main beam. Curved surfaces such as diaphragm, bladder or gall bladder and highly reflective interface such as with air are common conditions in which side lobe artifacts occur.

**Acoustic shadowing:** Appears as an area of low amplitude echoes (hypoechoic- to- anaechoic area) created by structures of high attenuation. It occurs as a result of nearly complete reflection or absorption of the sound. This artifact can be produced by gas or bone. Urinary calculi, barium and gall stones creates a strong clean acoustic shadow.

**Acoustic enhancement:** Also called through –transmission represents a localized increase of the echo amplitude occurring distal to a structure of low attenuation. This is commonly seen distal to the gall bladder and urinary bladder.

**Comets:** Artifacts produced on film that resemble comets. They are usually caused by rust particles adhering to film during development.

**Refraction:** It occurs when incident sound wave traverses tissues of different acoustic impedences. This may cause a reflector to be improperly displayed. Refraction between the spleen or liver and the adjacent fat and creates the duplication of the organ.

## Manipulating Artifacts

- Proper patient preparation with 12 hours fasting of filling the bladder and part of gastrointestinal tract with fluid.
- Choosing proper frequency of transducers for the organ of interest.
- Adjusting the power, gain and time-gain compensation setting correctly.
- Avoiding other electrical devices or radiofrequency signal interference.

## Indications for Ultrasonography (USG)

- Pregnancy diagnosis - as early as 14 days conceptual fluid is seen in equine, in canines as early as 20 days.
- Twin pregnancies, pregnancy losses, pseudopregnancy, Ovarian cysts and haematoma, ovarian tumours and infection.
- The organs which can be scanned usefully are liver, kidney, urinary bladder, spleen, uterus, ovaries, teat and udder.
- Merit of ultrasound is its ability to characterize internal parenchymal.

- Contrast radiography, angiography or exploratory laparotomy.
- Biopsy guidance for internal masses and cytocentesis (liver and kidney biopsies, pericardium and chest drainage).
- Bone heal monitoring.
- Cardiac evaluations (assessment of blood flow and supply).

## Strength of USG

- Non-invasive.
- Essentially non-toxic.
- Free from radiation hazards.
- Usually does not require general anaesthesia or sedation.
- Provide quick instant and dynamic visualization.
- Allows precise location of biopsy needle.
- Fetal viability.
- Real time scanning - see movement/motion (dynamic imaging).
- Relatively inexpensive compared to other modes of investigation, viz;CT or MRI.

## Weakness of USG

- Repetitive exam.
- Can't evaluate some extra abdominal structures (i.e. spine).
- High level of skill and experience is needed to acquire good-quality images and make accurate diagnosis.
- Must know anatomy very well.

## Therapeutic Applications

- Physical therapy and treatment of cancer.
- Cataract treatment by phacoemulsification.
- Break up kidney stones by lithotripsy.
- Interventional biopsy.
- Contrast-enhanced ultrasound.

## Imaging Approaches

In transabdominal scaning, the transducer is placed on ventral or lateral wall in small sized animal. In transrectal scanning, the transducer is taken per rectum under a rubber sleeve in large animals. In transurethral or transvaginal scanning special sector or radical endoluminal transducer are used to evaluate mucosal surface of urethra, bladder, vagina, cervix or uterus. Transthoracic scanning, is commonly used to scan heart and major vessels, lungs and dioaphragm. Sonoendoscopic transducers are also available which may allow transluminal evaluation of hollow visceral organs.

## Abdominal Ultrasonography

In abdominal scanning various abdominal organs are amenable to sonographic scanning: viz: hepatobiliary (hepatic size, abscess,cyst, tumour, cirrhosis, calculi, obstruction, infection of gall bladder and bile duct), spleen (abscess, tumour, infraction and splenic size), gastro-intestinal tract (foreign body, obstruction, tumors, mucosal pattern, peristalsis, gastric and intestinal emptying time), calculi in kidney and urinary bladder, hydronephrosis, bladder tumour, renal cortex and medulla are well visualized in sonographic scanning.

## Reproductive Ultrasonograpphy

Ultrasonography has been used to its fullest extent in animal reproduction to study ovarian follicular dynamics, pregnancy diagnosis, fetal well being including fetal sexing, ovum pick-up technology (OPU) and in the detection of reproductive diseases. The uterus appears as a well defined, tubular structure, with hypoechoic to anechoic lumen. Spectral, color flow and power Doppler imaging now facilitate physiologic interpretations of vascular dynamics over time. Pregnancy is diagnosed by the presence of anechoic vesicular conceptus. Sonography gives definite evidence of fetal viability in allowing visualization of fetal heartbeat, fetal development, fetal sexing and expected date of parturition. Program and formula are available to predict gestational age (GA) with parameters like gestational sac diameter (GSD), head diameter (HD), crown rump length (CRL)and body diameter (BD).

Gestational age in the dog:

$$GA= (6 \times GSD) + 20: GA=( 3 \times CRL) + 27.$$

Greater than 40 days:

$$GA= (15 \times HD) + 20: GA =(7 \times BD) + 29.$$

This method was less accurate for toy, miniature and giant breeds. A correction factor of +1day should be applied to the gestational age prediction for small body weight (<9 kg) bitches and -2 days for giant body weight (>40 kg) bitches.

**Ovum pick-up (OPU) technology:** Reproductive technologies like in *in-vivo* embryo production, production of cloned or transgenic animals and establishment of occyte banks have made a giant stride in recent years. The requirement of OPU comprised of an ultrasound scanner with a transvaginal transducer, needle guidance system and suction pump. Diseases of female reproduction tract like pyometra, mucometra, hydrometra, fetal mummification and ovarian tumours can be detected by ultrasonography. Physiological blood flow pattern of canine testis and prostate gland is documented sonographically. Testicular hypoplasia, benign prostatic, hyperplasis in canine are frequently diagnoses by ultrasonography.

**Cardiac ultrasonography/ Echocardiography:** When ultrasound is used to image the heart it is referred to as an echocardiogram, allows physicians to see detailed structures of the heart, including chamber size, heart function, the valves of the heart, as well as the pericardium. Echocardiography uses 2D, 3D and Doppler imaging to create pictures of the heart and visualize the blood flowing through each of the four heart valves. In emergency situations echocardiography is quick, easily accessible and able to be performed at the bedside making it the modality of choice for many physicians. Stress echocardiography is gaining ground as an evaluating tool for performance in racing horses.

**Limb ultrasonography:** Evaluation of tendons and ligaments of both forelimbs and hindlimbs is extensively used in racehorses to certify their fitness. It has been proved to be a superior imaging modality to detect adhesions, tearing and inflammatioin of these structures.

Besides, ultrasonography is being used for evaluation of endocrine glands, salivary glands, eyes, tissue healing, teat and udder.

## Ultrasound-guided Biopsy

Percutaneous biopsy of abdominal organs like liver, spleen, kidney, prostrate, abdominal mass, lesions *etc.* under ultrasound guidance is well documented. Biopsy site is prepared for aseptic intervention. The transducer is covered with a sterile sleeve and gel. Once a good sonographic image is the relevant organ is obtained, a biopsy needle is introduced through the abdominal wall, either via a clip-on guide at an angle of 15-30$^0$ to the transducer. The point of the needle can be directed precisely into the mass/lesion under guidance of the image on monitor. A variety of needle are available for biopsy collection. After sample collection the needle is withdrawn.

## Three Dimensional (3-D) Ultrasound (U/S)

Two-dimensional ultrasonography relies on the acquisition of images in multiple scan planes from which to build a mental 3 D images. Ultrasound waves are directed from multiple angles and waves are reflected back and captured, providing very detailed 3-dimensional images of the baby. Help in diagnosing certain conditions (such as a cleft lip) that may not be visible with 2D. Manipulated in a number of ways (rotation, zooming) to allow unprecedented examination of the U/S images.

## 2 types of 3-D U/S

- A) Featured based construction (surface rendering): provides a profile of the surface of the structure.
- B) Voxel based reconstruction (volume rending): each pixel acquired in the 2-D U/S images is placed into the proper 3-D.

## Four Dimensional (4-D) Ultrasound

The process of streaming 3-D images into live, real-time video of the baby. This allows viewers to see real-time motion. It is a newest form of 3-D and provides functional data in the 3-D. Applied in the echocardiography and neurosonology.

## Contrast Enhanced Ultrasonography

The field of diagnostic ultrasound is again on the cusp of major change. In the last decade, drug companies, ultrasound scanner manufacturers, and academic centers have invested manpower and funding in developing efficacious ultrasound contrast agents and new contrast-specific imaging modalities.

Ultrasound contrast medium exogenous substance that alter the echo amplitude in ultrasonography or Doppler ultrasound applications. Ultrasound (US) contrast agents (UCAs) are gas microbubbles encapsulated by albumin, lipids, polymer or surfactant shell. They are less than 10 μm in diameter and contain air or a low solubility gas such as perfluorocarbon. In diagnostic US, microbubbles injected intravenously increase the scattered echoes from vessels and flowing blood owing to their impedance mismatch, resonant and highly non-linear behaviours. At low mechanical index they produce linear backscatter enhancement. As the power is increased, bubbles scatter not only at the acoustic center frequency, but also at low multiples and simple fractions of the driving frequency. It is the detection of these non-linear components which is at the basis of contrast-specific modalities such as contrast harmonic and pulse inversion imaging and contrast Doppler, which are used to suppress tissue signals and enhance blood echo, particularly at the level of the smaller blood vessels.

- New Imaging tool – Must have the knowledge to understand how the image is formed. The benefits of contrast enhancement have long been recognized in CT and MRI, and it now appears that ultrasound contrast agents with both Doppler and gray-scale capabilities will soon be available to U.S. physicians. This will likely enhance the diagnostic usefulness of ultrasound. The systemic echo enhancement provided by ultrasound contrast agents should increase diagnostic confidence, especially in technically difficult cases with low image sensitivity. Moreover, contrast-specific imaging modalities, such as harmonic imaging and intermittent imaging, promise to put new tools for tumor diagnosis in the hands of clinicians.
- The microbubble contrast agents developed and introduced as safe and effective echo-enhancers in present-day clinical practice will open up new opportunities.
- The systemic echo enhancement provided by ultrasound contrast agents should increase diagnostic confidence, especially in technically difficult cases with low image sensitivity.

**Table 1** : Classification of Ultrasound contrast agents

| Microbubble | Gas | Stabilizing shell |
|---|---|---|
| *First generation, non-transpulmonary vascular* | | |
| Free microbubbles | Air | None |
| Echovist (SHU 454) | Air | None |
| *Second generation, transpulmonary vascular, short half-life (< 5 min)* | | |
| Albunex | Air | Albumin |
| Levovist (SHU 508 A) | Air | Palmitic acid |
| *Third generation, transpulmonary vascular, longer half-life (> 5 min)* | | |
| Aerosomes (Definity, MRX115, DMP115) | Perfluoropropane | Phospholipids |
| Echogen (QW3600) | Dodecafluoropentane | Surfactant |
| Optison (FSO 69) | Octafluoropropane | Albumin |
| PESDA | Perfluorobutane | Albumin |
| Quantison | Air | Albumin |
| QW7437 | Perfluorocarbon | Surfactant |
| Imavist (Imagent, AFO150) | Perfluorohexane | Surfactant |
| Sonovue (BR1) | Sulphur hexafluoride | Phospholipids |
| *Transpulmonary with organ-specific phase (liver, spleen)* | | |
| BR14 | Perfluorobutane | Phospholipids |
| Levovist (SHU 508 A) | Air | Palmitic acid |
| Sonavist (SHU 563 A) | Air | Cyanoacrylate |
| Sonazoid (NC100100) | Perfluorocarbon | Surfactant |

## General Features

There are a variety of microbubbles contrast agents. Microbubbles differ in their shell makeup, gas core makeup, and whether or not they are targeted.

- **Microbubble shell**: Selection of shell material determines how easily the microbubble is taken up by the immune system. A more hydrophilic material tends to be taken up more easily, which reduces the microbubble residence time in the circulation. This reduces the time available for contrast imaging. The shell material also affects microbubble mechanical elasticity. The more elastic the material, the more acoustic energy it can withstand before bursting. Currently, microbubble shells are composed of albumin, galactose, lipid, or polymers.

- **Microbubble gas core**: The gas core is the most important part of the ultrasound contrast microbubble because it determines the echogenicity. When gas bubbles are caught in an ultrasonic frequency field, they compress, oscillate, and reflect a characteristic echo- this generates the strong and unique sonogram in contrast-enhanced ultrasound. Gas cores can be composed of air, or heavy gases like perfluorocarbon, or nitrogen. Heavy gases are less water-soluble so they are less likely to leak out from the microbubble to impair echogenicity. Therefore, microbubbles with heavy gas cores are likely to last longer in circulation.

## Contrast Techniques

Many contrast-specific imaging modalities have been developed in recent years by academic researchers, ultrasound scanner manufacturers, and pharmaceutical companies, but most are variations, hybrids, or combinations of the following techniques.

i). Contrast-enhanced Doppler imaging. Colour amplitude imaging (CAI) shows the amplitude of the Doppler signal from moving blood flow, while colour Doppler imaging (CDI) depicts the mean frequency shifts of the Doppler signal (i.e., mean flow velocity). CAI is a relatively new ultrasound technique with increased dynamic range and flow sensitivity in comparison to conventional CDI.

ii). The sensitivity of Doppler ultrasound should be increased markedly in conjunction with the use of vascular contrast agents. Contrast harmonic imaging. CHI is a novel technique, opening the possibility of measuring blood perfusion or capillary blood flow-a clinically important task. It utilizes the nonlinear properties of contrast agents by transmitting at the fundamental frequency but receiving at the second harmonic.

iii). A bubble acts as a harmonic oscillator and contrast-enhanced echo signals thus contain significant energy components at higher harmonics, while tissue echoes do not. In other words, the nonlinearity of the contrast produces a “signature” that can be separated from tissue echoes and large vessel blood flow, allowing capillary blood flow (i.e., perfusion) to be calculated. Combined with the pulse inversion technique, CHI possesses not only a very high sensitivity to contrast agent but also a high spatial resolution, similar to the spatial resolution of conventional B-mode used in the same transmit-receive frequency band.

- *Intermittent imaging* : Contrast microbubbles can be destroyed by intense ultrasound and the scattered signal level can increase abruptly for a short time during microbubble destruction, resulting in sudden increase in echogenicity (acoustical "flash").

Intermittent imaging with high acoustic output utilizes the unique property of contrast microbubbles to improve blood-to-tissue image contrast by imaging intermittently at very low frame rates instead of the conventional 30 frames per second. The frame rate is usually reduced to about one frame per second, or it is synchronized with cardiac cycles so that enough contrast microbubbles can flow into the imaging site where most microbubbles have been destroyed by the previous acoustic pulse. Because bubbles are destroyed by ultrasound, controlling the delay time between frames produces images whose contrast emphasizes regions with rapid blood flow or regions with high or low blood volume.

## Applications of Contrast-Enhanced Ultrasound

Untargeted contrast-enhanced ultrasound is currently applied in echocardiography. Targeted contrast-enhanced ultrasound is being developed for a variety of medical applications.

**Untargeted CEUS:** Like Optison and Levovist are currently used in echocardiography.

- **Organ Edge Delineation**: Microbubbles can enhance the contrast at the interface between the tissue and blood. A clearer picture of this interface gives the clinician a better picture of the structure of an organ. Tissue structure is crucial in echocardiograms, where a thinning, thickening, or irregularity in the heart wall indicates a serious heart condition that requires either monitoring or treatment.
- **Blood Volume and Perfusion**: Contrast-enhanced ultrasound holds the promise for (1) evaluating the degree of blood perfusion in an organ or area of interest and (2) evaluating the blood volume in an organ or area of interest. When used in conjunction with Doppler ultrasound,

microbubbles can measure myocardial flow rate to diagnose valve problems. And the relative intensity of the microbubble echoes can also provide a quantitative estimate on blood volume.

## Targeted CEUS

- **Inflammation**: In inflammatory diseases such as Crohn's disease, atherosclerosis, and even heart attacks, the inflamed blood vessels specifically express certain receptors like VCAM-1, ICAM-1, E-selectin. If microbubbles are targeted with ligands that bind these molecules, they can be used in contrast echocardiography to detect the onset of inflammation. Early detection allows the design of better treatments.
- **Cancer**: Cancer cells also express a specific set of receptors, mainly receptors that encourage angiogenesis, or the growth of new blood vessels. If microbubbles are targeted with ligands that bind receptors like VEGF, they can non-invasively and specifically identify areas of cancers.
- **Gene Delivery**: Vector DNA can be conjugated to the microbubbles. Microbubbles can be targeted with ligands that bind to receptors expressed by the cell type of interest. When the targeted microbubble accumulates at the cell surface with its DNA payload, ultrasound can be used to burst the microbubble. The force associated with the bursting may temporarily permeablize surrounding tissues and allow the DNA to more easily enter the cells.
- **Drug Delivery**: Drugs can be incorporated into the microbubble's lipid shell. The microbubble's large size relative to other drug delivery vehicles like liposomes may allow a greater amount of drug to be delivered per vehicle. By targeted the drug-loaded microbubble with ligands that bind to a specific cell type, microbubble will not only deliver the drug specifically, but can also provide verification that the drug is delivered if the area is imaged using ultrasound.

## Advantages of Contrast-Enhanced Ultrasound

On top of the strengths mentioned in the medical sonography entry, contrast-enhanced ultrasound adds these additional advantages.

- The body is 73% water, and therefore, acoustically homogeneous. Blood and surrounding tissues have similar echogenicities, so it is also difficult to clearly discern the degree of blood flow, perfusion, or the interface between the tissue and blood using traditional ultrasound.
- Ultrasound imaging allows real-time evaluation of blood flow.
- Ultrasonic molecular imaging is safer than molecular imaging modalities such as radionuclide imaging because it does not involve radiation.
- Alternative molecular imaging modalities, such as MRI, PET, and SPECT are very costly. Ultrasound, on the other hand, is very cost-efficient and widely available.
- Since microbubbles can generate such strong signals, a lower intravenous dosage is needed, micrograms of microbubbles are needed compared to milligrams for other molecular imaging modalities such as MRI contrast agents.
- Targeting strategies for microbubbles are versatile and modular. Targeting a new area only entails conjugating a new ligand.

## Disadvantages of Contrast-Enhanced Ultrasound

In addition to the weaknesses mentioned in the medical sonography entry, contrast-enhanced ultrasound suffers from the following disadvantages:

- Microbubbles don't last very long in circulation. They have low circulation residence times because they either get taken up by immune system cells or get taken up by the liver or spleen even when they are coated with PEG.
- Ultrasound produces more heat as the frequency increases, so the ultrasonic frequency must be carefully monitored.
- Microbubbles burst at low ultrasound frequencies and at high mechanical indices (MI), which is the measure of the acoustic power output of the ultrasound imaging system. Increasing MI increases image quality, but there are tradeoffs with microbubble destruction. Microbubble destruction could cause local microvasculature ruptures and hemolysis.
- Targeting ligands can be immunogenic, since current targeting ligands used in preclinical experiments are derived from animal culture.

- Low targeted microbubble adhesion efficiency, which means a small fraction of injected microbubbles bind to the area of interest. This is one of the main reasons that targeted contrast-enhanced ultrasound remains in the preclinical development stages.

## Magnetic Resonance Imaging (MRI)

MRI is the technique in which the protons of body tissues are subjected to an artificially created strong magnetic field. MRI scanner uses powerful magnets to polarize and excite hydrogen nuclei (single proton ) in water molecules in tissue, producing a detectable signal which is spatially encoded resulting in images of the body. Their ability to return to the origin spin is gauged by computer device.

## Principle

Basic principle of MRI is that certain atomic nuclei will absorb and remit radio waves when placed in a strong magnetic field. Radio waves remitted can be used to construct a diagnostic anatomic image through a computer -assisted technique termed MRI. In brief, MRI, involves the use of three kinds of electromagnetic field; a very strong static magnetic field to polarize the hydrogen nuclei, called the static field; a weaker time varying field for encoding, called the gradient field, and a weak radio-frequency field to produce measureable single.

## Application of MRI

- FLAIR (fluid light attenuation inversion recovery) sequence useful for determining difference between normal and edematous tissue fluid.
- To distinguish pathological tissue from normal tissue.
- Provides accurate and detailed anatomic images with a good contrast and spatial resolution (ability to distinguish between to arbitrarily similar but not identical tissue).

## Advantages of MRI

- MRI is a highly sensitive and non- invasive technique (does not use ionizing radiation and therefore not associated with health hazards).

- Can be used for diagnosis of brain and nervous system disorders, spinal disorders, cardiovascular diseases, osteochondrosis, neoplastic mass and joint diseases.
- It has the ability to image in any plane.
- MRI contrast materials have a very low or no incidence of side effects.
- MRI involves a relatively short examination time.
- MRI can eliminate the need for biopsy or exploratory surgery in some cases, and can detect problem that have been hidden on prior tests.
- MRI offers an exceptional view of internal organs. The high sensitivity of MRI, combined with 3-D viewing, produces diagnostic images of outstanding clarity.

## Disadvantage

- MRI system are very, expensive to purchase, and therefore this technique is reserved for few selected cases.
- Needs specially constructed rooms without any metallic structures.
- Needs expertise to perform the examination and interpret the results.
- The machine makes a tremendous amount of noise (like a continual, rapid hammering) during a scan.
- Orthopaedic hardware (screws, plates,artificial joints) in the area of a scan can cause severe artifacts (distortions) on the images due to singnificant alteration in the main magnetic field.
- MRI is not indicated in acutely traumatized patients, since life support systems cannot be safely used in the magnetic field.

## Magnetic Resonance Spectroscopy (MRS)

Emerging as a diagnostic imaging tool capable of analyzing phosphorus or hydrogen content of the imaged tissue. A non-invasive characterization of imaged tissue can be derived and will allow the neuroncologists to make more rapid diagnosis and initiate the appropriate therapy. It is not only differentiating tumor from infarction, but also for detecting tumor cell type. *In-vivo* brain metabolism can also be studies using MR spectroscopy.

## Advantage

Provide detailed chemical information about the region.

## Functional Magnetic Resonance Imaging (fMRI)

fMRI measures the signal changes in the brain that are due to changing neural activity. It is a revolutionary extension of MRI technology applied to the study of human brain function. fMRI is non-invasive and offers much higher spatial and temporal resolution than previous brain mapping techniques, combine with exceptional anatomic localization.

## Nuclear Scintigraphy (NS) or Nucler Medicine (NM)

Nuclear scintigraphic imaging is a highly sensitive advanced procedure which done by injecting a radioactive isotope intravenously and are used to detect functional abnormalities of the body system. Usually Technetium 99M is used. This is a gamma-rays emitting isotope, and when combined with phosphate compounds, it localizes within bones, greater in the regions of high turnover or regions of increased circulation thus producing "hotspots". These hotspots are usually indicators of an abnormality. A gamma camera is required to detect gamma ray emitted by the isotops.

## Principle of NS

Is based on the use of pharmaceutical, which after entry into the blood streams gets localized in a particular tissue or organ. Before the pharmaceutical is injected it is labeled with a radioisotope. Thus localization of the isotope can then be detected by using detector or camera due to emission of gamma rays from the area of interest. A computer system is usually attached to the camera for gathering data and its display and quantification. The scan appears as a image formed of dots. The interpretation is based on the appearance of increased (hot spots) or decreased (cold spots) radioactivity regions.The physiological or pathological disorder can be easily detected.

**Uses:** Has been used to detect functional disorders of kidney, liver, GI tract, Lung ventilation and perfusion, thyroid, bone, bone tumors, *etc.*

**Disadvantage:** High cost, safety measures, etiological non-specificity and difficult in interpretation especially in skeletal system.

## Scientigraphy Positron Emission Tomography (PET) or Single Photon Emission Computed Tomography (SPECT)

Techniques allows qualitative and quantitative measurement of physiologic processes as well as alterations secondary to various disease states. With the use of specific radioligands, molecular pathways and pharmacokinetic processes can be investigated.

## Diagnostic Thermography

Thermography is the measurement of temperature variations at the body surface and thus is the pictorial representation of the surface temperature of an object. Thermography is a non-contact, non-invasive technique that detects surface heat emitted as infrared radiation. Variations in heat are represented by different colours. The hottest areas are white and red while the cooler regions are represented by the darker blues and black. Interpretation of the colour pattern is thought to contribute to the diagnosis of many disorders.

A medical thermogram representing the surface temperatures of skin, makes it useful for the detection of inflammation as heat is one of the cardinal signs of inflammation.

## Endoscopy/Laparoscopy

Endoscopy (endo=inside, scope=vision, means looking inside) is the visualization of the interior of a body cavity through an endoscope for diagnostic and therapeutic purposes. Unlike most other medical imaging devices, endoscopes are inserted directly into the organ. It is a non-surgical procedure used to examine a patient's hollow organs. An endoscope is a medical device consisting of a long, thin, flexible (or rigid) tube which has a light and a video camera. The pictures captured by the camera are viewed on a colour TV monitor. During an upper endoscopy, an endoscope is easily passed through the mouth and throat and into the esophagus allowing the doctor to view the esophagus, stomach, and upper part of the small intestine. Similarly, endoscopes can be passed into the large intestine (colon) through the rectum to examine this area of the intestine. This procedure is called colonoscopy. The whole endoscopy is recorded so that doctors can check it again.

**Endoscopy can be used for any of the following:**

- Investigation of lesions, such as in the digestive system.
- Confirmation of a diagnosis, most commonly by performing a biopsy to check for conditions such as bleeding *etc.*
- Giving treatment, such as cauterization of a bleeding vessel, widening a narrow esophagus, clipping off a polyp or removing a foreign object.

There are many different kinds of endoscopy. Here are the names of some of them and where they look.

- Arthroscopy: joints.
- Bronchoscopy: lungs.
- Colonoscopy and sigmoidoscopy: large intestine.
- Cystoscopy and ureteroscopy: urinary system.
- Laparoscopy: abdomen or pelvis.
- Upper gastrointestinal endoscopy: esophagus and stomach.

## Interventional Imaging

Is a new medical sub-especialty, which utilizes minimally - invasive image guided procedures to diagnose and treat diseases in nearly every organ system. The concept behind interventional imaging is to diagnose and treat patients using the least invasive techniques currently available in order to minimize risk to the patient and improve health outcomes. Using X-rays, ultrasound, CT, MRI and other imaging modalities, interventional radiologist obtain images which are then used to direct interventional instruments throughout the body. These procedures are performed using needle and narrow called catheters, rather than by making larger incisions into the body as in traditional surgery.

Many conditions that once required surgery can now be treated non-surgically by interventional radiologist. By minimizing the physical trauma to the patient, peripheral interventions can reduce infection rates and recovery time, as well as shorten hospital stays. Interventional radiologist Charles Dotter, known as the "Father of Interventional Radiology" for pioneering the technique, was nominated for the Noble prize in Physiology or Medicine in 1978.

# Chapter - 23

# Principles of Radiation Therapy

Radiation therapy is the delivery of ionizing radiation to a specific body areas with the goal of obtaining maximum lesion control with minimal complication. Radiation therapy is based on the fact that ionizing radiation is lethal to the cells, particularly rapidly dividing ones. Normal cells in the irradiated area may be as sensitive to ionizing radiation as tumor cells. Therefore, the normal tissue response limits the amount of ionizing radiation that can be tolerated by the patient. Effective use of radiation therapy requires an understanding of the physics of the radiation used and normal cellular and tumor biology as it relates to radiation therapy as well as an appreciation of the clinical application of veterinary radiation therapy.

In 1906-1912, R. Eberlein was first to report radiation therapy in veterinary practice. In veterinary medicine, radiation therapy has been practiced to a minor role in the treatment of cancer. In case of ruminants even this use is very limited, mainly due to non-availability of facility, lack of technical know-how and the expenditure involved. Only sporadic cases and reports are available on the use of radiotherapy in the management of bovine tumors. A success rate of 90% has been reported following irradiation of squamous cell carcinoma of the eye, eyelid and face using gold-198 in cattle.

Nevertheless, as awareness to this form of therapy among veterinarians heightens and the treatment is increased in its efficacy by the development of newer techniques, as well as an increase in the number of trained veterinary radiotherapists and radiologists, the situation will indeed improve and newer uses for radiotherapy in combination with surgery and chemotherapy will become more common.

## Radiotherapy Terminology

**Radiosensitivity:** Refers to susceptibility of the cells or tissue to the killing effect of absorbed radiation.

**Radioresponsive:** Is the degree to which a normal or neoplastic tissue visibility changes during or after radiotherapy.

**Radiocurability:** Is the two-year patient survival after radiotherapy without further progress of the neoplasm and subsequent metastasis.

**Tumor lethal dose-** It is that dose of radiation that produces lethal effect on tumor. It also depends on type of tumor.

**Normal tissue tolerance dose-** Radiation dose that does not produce any pathological lesions to normal tissues. It is the deciding factor to determine therapy doses. It depends on types of cells.

**Therapeutic ratio:** It is the ratio of normal tissue tolerance dose to tumor lethal dose. Higher the therapeutic ratio more is the efficacy of radiotherapy.

**Tissue tolerance to radiotherapy:** Limitations in controlling malignancy or benign neoplasm by radiations is that we have to do it with minimal normal tissue complications.

## Indications for Radiotherapy

- Radiotherapy is indicated in localized solid neoplasms that cannot be excised completely. Usually not indicated if neoplasm has the potential of high incidence of metastasis.
- When surgery is expected to or has failed.
- When regional or distant metastasis has not occurred.
- When radical surgery is unable to remove whole of the neoplasm.
- When bulk of neoplasm require reduction in size so that can be removed surgically.

**Disadvantage:** Because of the potential side effects, debilitated patient should not be subjected to radiotherapy.

## DO's before Radiotherapy

- Patient evaluation: Through clinical examination of the patient.
- Complete blood count (CBC), urine analysis,
- Radiograph of the primary site of the tumor, radiograph of thorax and abdomen to check evidence of metastasis.

## Mechanism of action of Radiation

Two theories are postulated

A. **Direct or Target theory:** The theory proposes that radiant energy acts by a direct hit on the target molecules configuration of the molecule and thus damage to the cell. The DNA molecule is the most important target of radiation in the cell, especially linkages and bonds within the DNA molecule. Depending upon the radiosensitivity of the tissue, dose and duration of radiation is computed and there are three principle effects on the DNA molecule:

1). *Genetic damage-* If damage occurs in germ cells, response is observed in the next generation.

2). *Production of cancer-* If the proper dose is not used upto a particular period, there will be derangement of the DNA resulting in abnormal metabolic activity causing production of malignant disease.

3). *Cell death-* DNA plays an important role in cell division and is also important for maintaining life of cell. When radiations damage DNA, cell division is interfered. This explains the death of cancer by ionizing radiations. So radiations can cause cancer or can treat cancer.

B. **Indirect theory:** This theory proposes that radiant energy exerts its effects by producing free 'hot ' radicals such as peroxides within the cell that damage the specific target. Water molecule is the major constituent of the cell. $H_2O$ H-, OH- or unstable $HO_2$ and $H_2O_2$, these are highly unstable molecule and react amongst themselves and other solutes within the solution thus producing crucial biological damage to cell thus causing cell death.

## Planning for Radiotherapy

Radiotherapy is not given by a single dose, rather it is given in divided dosed spread over a period of time (fractioned therapy). In veterinary practice, therapy is usuaully in 10 -12 fractions of a radiation dose of 4-5 Gy each time, usually three per weeks. This is done through 4 R's of radiotherapy:

1. *Reoxygenation:* Oxygenated cells are killed earlier, more oxygen become available to hypoxic radioresistant cells to make them radiosensitive.
2. *Repopulation:* The ability of tumor cells to repopulate is slower than normal tissue following radiotherapy.
3. *Redistribution:* Exposes the cells within the cell cycle at a phase when they are radiosensitive.
4. *Repair:* Repair of most normal cells take place faster than that of tumour cells during the gap period of fractioned therapy.

## Methods of Radiotherapy

## A. Teletherapy

Teletherapy, or external radiation therapy, is the use of radiation source at a distance from the patient/tumor. Electronic teletherapeutic machines commonly X-rays in the orthovoltage or supervoltage energy range. It is of four types:

1. *Superficial X-ray therapy:* Orthovoltage machines are used to treat superficial lesions or tumors that have been surgically exposed. It is given with energy range of 60-100 Kev.
2. *Deep X-ray therapy:* Supervoltage X-ray machine with the energy range of 200-300 keV are called linear accelerators used to treat tumors that are deep within the body or that are closely associated with bony structures.
3. *Supervoltage therapy:* It can be provided through i). X-ray machines having linear accelerator (1 Mev to 20 Mev) or Betatron (20 Mev to 100 Mev) or cyclotron. ii).Through isotopic X-ray machine with Cobalt or Cesium in a sealed form.
4. *Particulate Beam Therapy:* Electron (e), Neutron (N) or Proton (P) beam can also be used as a mode of teletherapy.

## B. Brachytherapy

It is the therapeutic use of radioisotopes in the form of surface applicators, with in wires, needles, seeds or grains etc. remains in touch or implanted with the tumor tissues. The methods are

1. **Interstitial Brachytherapy:** When the sources or radiation are within the interstitium of the tumor e.g. Gold (Au) -198, cobalt (Co)-60. etc.

   *Advantages:* Is short half life, removable continuous low dose irradiation of the tumour and high total doses obtained within the tumor. Implantation requires a single anesthetic procedure and ospitalization time is less. Normal tissue is least affected.

   *Disadvantages:* Implantation is invasive, often a difficult procedure. Special training is required.

2. **Pliesotherapy (Surface brachytherapy):** Is used to treat small, superficial lesions. Use of Strontium (Sr) -90 is frequently used for superficial lesions in the management of eosinophilic grnuloma, lick granuloma, corneal vascularisation and superficial squamous cell carcinoma.

3. **Systemic brachytherapy:** Is systemic administration of radioisotopes in which the radioisotopes become concentrated in either the tumor or the organ of interest. Two isotopes that can be systemically administered are Iodine (I)-131 and phosphorus (P)-32. The therapy is indicated for hyperthyroidism and selected cases of thyroid carcinoma.

4. Sometimes the radioactive source is delivered to the tumour through tubes and then withdrawn—an approach called remote brachytherapy.

## Complication of Radiotherapy

Generally 2 types of complications are observed: Immediate and Latent.

Immediate complications: are those, which are observed within minutes or days after irradiation. They include:

- Epilation (hair loss),
- Moist desquamation of skin,
- Skin erythema.

- Chromosome aberration,
- Hematological depression.

Latent complications: When complications are not observable within months or years and occur after a long gap of time.

They include:

- Leukemia,
- Cancer, life span shortening and
- Lethal genes in coming generations.

Complications also depend upon the area to be irradiated.

In case of ophthalmic neoplasm irradiation, the effects can be in form of conjunctivitis, keratitis, cataract *etc.* These complications are not life threatening but may impair vision.

In case of radiotherapy of bone, complications may include fracture, septic osteo radio-necrosis and sarcoma formation.

# Chapter - 24

# Radiation Hazards and Safety

It has been well established that the risk of health problems rises as the amount of radiation exposure increases. All types of radiation produce changes in the living tissues. The resultant cellular injury causes physiological and pathological changes leading to "Radiation sickness". The radiation effects may be somatic or genetic. Somatic effects are harmful to a person in his lifetime whereas genetic effects affect generations. Radiation may cause changes in complex molecular systems of living cells, primarily in following two ways :-

1. **Direct interactions:** These appear when molecules of the body are modified due to absorption of energy of the incident photons of X-rays or any other radiation.
2. **Indirect interactions:** These appear due to the damage caused by the product of radiation decomposition (Radiolysis) of water and other solutes of the body.

*Direct interactions/effects:* Following three important mechanisms brings these about,

1. **Thermalization:** This is a process where incident radiations (X-ray photons) agitate the living macromolecules in a non-destructive manner and in the process transfer their kinetic energy and thereby increase the temperature of the molecular system. Of course if the temperature of the material becomes too high, complex organic molecules may break apart (*i.e.* the material gets "cooked") resulting in destruction.

2. **Excitation:** This is a process whereby the incident radiation while traversing through the tissue force bound electrons to be "knocked" free from their parent atoms or molecules. These free electrons are then available to interact with other atoms and molecules within the irradiated system. Generally however the free electrons are quickly captured and their energy added to the overall thermal energy of the system with little or no other effect.

3. **Ionization:** This is a process whereby molecules absorb sufficient energy from radiation to break their molecular bonds. This causes the direct modification or destruction of complex molecules. Covalent bonds and ionic bonds, the bonds between the atoms that form simple inorganic molecules such as sodium chloride (common table salt) have binding energies of about 2 to 5eV, about one half the strength of the ionizing energies of individual atoms. Organic molecules, many of which are important in cell biology, have bond energies of about 0.04 to 0.3eV and are typically referred to as "weak bonds".

**Two types of exposure to ionizing radiation:**

1. **Acute exposure:** Appears quickly (days or weeks) and a minimum dose of 100 rads is needs. A single, generally accidental, exposure to a high dose of radiation during a relatively short period of time which produces severe biological effects very soon after exposure radiation sickness is known as " acute radiation sickness" (ARS), is a serious illness that occurs when the entire body or most of it receives a high dose of radiation, usually over a short period of time. People exposed to radiation will get ARS only if: the radiation dose was high (doses from medical procedures such as chest X-rays are too low to cause ARS, however doses from radiation therapy to treat cancer may be high enough to cause some ARS symptoms), the radiation was penetrating that is able to reach internal organs, the persons entire body or most of it, received the dose, and the radiation was received in a short time, usually within minutes.

2. **Chronic exposure:** Is continuous or intermittent exposure to low levels of radiation over a long period of time. Chronic exposure may produce only effects that can be observed some time following initial exposure. These may include genetic

effects and other effects such as cancer, precancerous lesions, benign tumors, cataracts, skin changes, and congenital defects. Unsafe conditions if access interlocks are not working, shielding has been damaged, new X-ray tube was installed, viewing glass is cracked or a fixed X-ray device has been moved. The health effects of chronic exposure if they occur may not be apparent until many years often upto 20 years after the period of exposure.

**Radiation sensitivity of different body cells:** Radiation sensitivity refers to the loss of reproductive capability of the proliferating cells. Regularly proliferating cells are more sensitive. Therefore, stems cells of haemopoietic systems and cells of the gut, skin & testes are highly radiosensitive whereas, cells of nerve and muscles are relatively radio-resistant. Different body cells in order of decreasing radio-sensitivity : Lymphoid cells > Epithelial cells of the small intestine > Haemopoietic cells > Germinal cells > Epithelial cells of the skin > Connective tissue cells > Cartilage and growing bone cells > Cells of the brain and spinal cord > Cells of the skeletal muscles and mature bone.

## Exposure Terminology

## Measurement of Radiation (Unit)

**Electron volt (eV):** Which measures the energy of an X-ray, is called Electron volt (eV). Amount of energy gained by an electron as it accelerated by a potential difference of one volt. It is also expressed in thousand electron volts (keV). 1000eV = keV(Kilo electron volt)

There are several units used to measure levels of ionizing radiation

1. **Roentgen (R)** - It is the quantity of X-rays or gamma radiation, which produces one electrostatic unit (2.08 x 109 pairs/$cm^3$) in 1c.c. of dry air after its ionization at $0^0$C and 760 mm Hg. Not used for particle radiation. This unit(R) does not describe dose to tissue. The unit rad (Radiation absorbed dose) is used as a unit of absorbed dose following exposure to any type of ionizing radiation.

2. **Rad (radiation absorbed dose):** One rad is equal to the radiation necessary to deposit energy of 100 ergs in 1 gm. of irradiated material (100 ergs/gm.). Used for all types of ionizing radiation.

3. **Rem (Roentgen equivalent man):** Rem is the amount used to express the dose equivalent that results from exposure to ionizing radiation.

One rem = rad x quality factor.

The quality factor for X-rays and gamma rays is one.

4. **Sievert (Sv):** Sv is used to define a rem. It is becoming a commonly used unit to measure equivalent absorbed dose. The units of measurement are Sv (1 Sv= 100 rem).

5. **Gray (Gy) :** One joule of energy per kg of absorbed material. 1Gy=100 rads.

**Dose retemeter:** Any instrument which measure radiation dose rate.

**Dosimeter:** Instrument to detect and measure accumulated radiation exposure. In common use, a pencil size ionization chamber with a self-reading electrometer used for personnel monitoing.

**Thermoluminescent dosimeter:** A dosimeter made of certain crystalline material which is capable of both storing a fraction of absorbed ionizing radiation and releasing this energy in the form of visible photons when heated. The amount of light released can be used as a measure of radiation exposure to these crystals.

**Geiger-Mueller counter:** Highly sensitive, gas filled,radiation-measuring devices, operates at voltage sufficiently high to produce avalanche ionization and the pulse produces is independent of the number of ions formed in the gas by the primary ionizing particle.

**Film badge:** A packet of photographic film used for the approximate measurement of radiation exposure for personnel monitoring purposes. The badge may contain two or more films of differing sensitivity and it may contain filters which shield parts of the film from certain types of radiation.

**Relative biological effectiveness (RBE):** A factor used in radiobiology to compare the biological effectiveness of absorbed radiation doses (that is rad) due to different types of ionizing radiation, more specifically. It is the experimentally determined ratio of an absorbed dose of a reference radiation required to produce an identical biological effect in a particular experimental organism or tissue.

**Quality factor (Q):** The linear energy transfer dependent factor by which absorbed doses are multiplied to obtain a quantity that expresses, on common scale for all ionizing radiations, the effectiveness of the absorbed dose.

**Isotopic tracer:** The isotopic or non-natural mixture of isotopes of an element which may be incorporated into a sample to make observation in the course of that element, alone or in combination, through a chemical, biological or physical process.

**Maximum permissible dose (MPD):** MPD is the dose equivalent that persons are allowed to receive in a stated period of time. It is this dose that helps to determine whether procedures and equiptment in use are adequate to provide the degree of protection to the worker that is required.

**MPD for veterinarians and radiographic staff:** Body part -5000m rem; Whole body, gonads, bone- 100 m rem;Marrow, lens of the eye- 1500 m rem; Hand, forearms and feet- 75000 m rem.

## Principles of Radiation Safety

Various safety measures are always incorporated into X-ray machine and accelerators to protect the operators, including shielding and interlocks. All persons working in or near an area where X-rays are being generated must observe proper safety precautions. X-rays can be dangerous. As there of lack is physical sensation and delay in onset of some of the tissue damaging effects that can be caused by high doses or prolonged exposure to ionizing radiation. Long-term overexposure to radiation may result in loss of hair, redness and inflammation of the skin, blood count change, cell atrophy (wasting away), ulcerations, sterility, genetic damage, cancer, leukemia, and death.

NEVER stand in the path of the central X-ray beam during exposure.

NEVER hold the X-ray film packet in the patient's mouth during exposure.

NEVER hold the tube head or the tube head cylinder of the X-ray machine during exposure carrier at least what number of feet from the tube head.

The general principle of safety from X-ray radiation is simply to avoid unnecessary exposure to X-rays. The major goal of radiation safety is to ensure that all radiation exposures are as low as reasonably achievable (ALARA). This can be done in three (TDS) ways:

*Time (T):* Reducing the time one is exposed to X-rays. A worker receives a dose of radiation directly proportional to the amount of time spent in a radiation field. Thus reducing the time by one-half will reduce the radiation dose received by one-half. Operators should always work quickly and spend as little time as possible around the equipment while it is operating.

*Distance (D):* Increasing the distance from the source. Obviously greater the distance from a radiation producing machine lesser will be the radiatioin exposure. The radiation exposure lowers as the inverse square of the distance from the radiation source. That is 2x the distance; the exposure would b ¼ of the exposure at the original distance (1/2).

*Shilding (S):* Use of protective clothing containing lead. The best and easy way of reducing radiation exposure is to place a shielding between the machine operator and the source of radiation. Lead is commonly used for shielding. For low energy X-rays other materials including thick plastic, aluminium and wood can be used. Concrete, compacted earth and iron are often used for accelerator shielding. Shielding for protection against X-rays is of two categories:

1. **Source shielding:** Is a lead shield that enclosed the X-ray tube. This type of shilding is needed to protect against leakage which is all radiation except for the useful X-ray beam.
2. **Structural shielding:** Is designed to protect personnel from the useful X-ray beam and scattered X-rays. It encloses both the X-ray tube and space in which the irradiated subject is located. It can be a lead lined box, shilding in room walls or ceilings placed between the operator and the subject. Plastic and wood have a density of about 10% that of lead hence the thickness of these shields needs to be considerably greater.

## Protective/Safety Practice

1. Radiography should only be undertaken where there is definite justification to do so.
2. Exposure to personnel should be kept to a minimum.
3. Increase the distance between radiation source and personnel. Only the minimum required personnel should be present inside X-ray room during exposure.
4. The patient should preferably be restrained by chemical methods and not manually. A cassette holding device should be used whenever possible.
5. The operator should be behind shielding screen or at least 6 feet away from X-ray source.
6. **Use of protective barriers:** to minimize the risk of radiation reaching the operator and assistant.

Protective barriers are necessary to protect oneself from scattered radiation.

*Protective screen:* Screen made up of lead or painted with lead with glass pan in upper 1/3rd and is held in between the X-ray plant and control panel and protect operator from radiation hazards.

*Mobile protecting chair:* Chair with lead screen in front of about 3′ height and comes under protective equipment.

*Lead aprons:* Made up of lead rubber covered with cloth, or plastic impregnated with lead lining minimum of 0.25 mm and maximum of 0.5 mm equivalent for voltage up to 100 kV. Available in different sizes and types. a) Single sides having front is covered with apron and are strapped on back of the body. b) In double sided apron is on both side and fasten at side. c) Coat type they are like coat type. They are meant for protecting body against scattered radiation.

*Lead gloves and sleeves:* The individuals handling the animals for X-rays should wear protective gloves made up of lead rubber having lead lining minimum of 0.33 mm and maximum of 0.5 mm equivalent for voltage up to 100 kV.

*Lead goggles:* For protection of the eye while using fluoroscreening against the direct and the scattered radiations having lead equivalency of 0.25-2mm.

*Gonad and Thyroid shields:* Available in three different sizes of large, medium and small and having lead equivalency of 0.5 mm.

1. X-ray room and shielding equipments-
   - The wall of X-ray room should be of at least 22 cms thick concrete.
   - The wall should be painted with radiation absorbent paint.
   - When there is possibility of X-ray beam consistently directed horizontally, the wall should have a lead lining sandwiched between plywood.
   - Whenever possible X-ray operator should be in a lead shielded cabin during exposure.
2. Use of optimal exposure factors and reduction of unnecessary radiography. Different radiographic accessories which reduce exposure factors (e.g. intensifying screens) should be used along with correct exposure factors. Radiography should not be done just because of owner's wish; a radiologist should decide its necessity.

3. Always use a collimator and always use the smallest possible aperture that will cover the anatomic area of interest.
4. Use of radiation monitoring devices: Personnel exposure detection meter / dosemeters should be worn by all personnel involved in radiography to record any radiation to which they are exposed. A busy radiographer should get his badge checked every month; a less busy radiographer may get it checked every three month.
5. Consideration for sex and age of the personnel involved: Person under 18 years of age should not be involved in radiographic work because of the sensitivity of their growing tissues. Similarly due to sensitivity of ova and embryos at certain stage of development, pregnant, potentially pregnant and women during menstrual cycle should avoid X-ray work.
6. Engineering safety controls: include shielding and warning systems installed to prevent over exposure to radiation. The X-ray head is always shielded, the beam path is often enclosed for some types of machines such a X-ray diffraction machines and ideally there is shielding in place to absorb radiation scattered by the irradiated subject.
7. An interlock is a device for precluding access to an aera with a radiation hazard by either preventing entry while the machine is operating or shutting off the machine if entry is attempted.
8. Log book maintenance is a must every time the machine used which should include information such as operators name, date, procedure performed, operating parameters (kV, mA).
9. The doors to all rooms containing a radiation producing machine must be labeled with a "Caution –X-ray" sign or "Caution Radiation area" in addition to a label on the machine: "This equipment produces radiation when energized".
10. Personnel associated with the operation of X-ray machine shall be provided with individual radiatioin monitoring badges. For availing personnel monitoring services, please contact Head Personnel Monitoring Service Section, Health, Safety and Environment Group, Bhabha Atomic Research Centre, CT and CRS Building, Anushaktinagar, Mumbai-400094.

11. All persons working in the X-ray unit must be provided with radiation dosimeters.

## Radiation Dosimetry

- Radiation dosimeter are devices that measure the accumulated dose of radiation-thermoluminescent dosimeters (TLD) to be worn at collar level. Ring bages are also used by some operators. The dosimeter has to be worn by the person to whom it is assigned. When not worn the dosimeter must be stored well away from radiation source since they are intended to measure the dose to the person and not to the room.
- Area monitor dosimeter badges are posted in rooms containing a radiation producing machine to measure the ambient level of radiation in potentially affected areas as that radiation might impact persons in nearby uncontrolled areas such as offices and conference rooms.

# Chapter - 25

# Glossary

**A, an:** Prefixes signifying without, lack of, *e.g.* atypical is not characteristic of type.

**ab, abs:** Prefixes signifying away from, departure, eg abduct is to draw away from median plane or axis.

**Absorb :** To suck in, as in a sponge; to assimilate fluids or other substances from skin.

**Absorbed dose:** The amount of energy deposited by ionizing radiationin a unit mass of tissue. It is expressed in units of joule per kilogram (J/kg), and called "Gray" (Gy).

**Absorption unsharpness:** The unsharpness in the image due to variations in absorption throughout a three-dimensional structure, caused by the particular shape of that structure. For example, a spherical object projects "unsharp" edges onto film.

**Absorption:** As applied to radiography, the act of attenuating an X-ray beam. Tissues of different densities have differing numbers of X-ray photons and therefore appear relatively "blacker" (less dense) or "white" (denser) on an X-ray film. Lead, which is denser than most materials, is one of the best absorber of X-rays.

**Activator:** Chemical, usually acetic acid in the fixer and sodium carbonate in the developer, used to neutralise the developer and swell the gelatin.

**Activity(radioactivity):** The property of certain nuclides of emitting radiation by spontaneous transformation of their nuclei. Various units of (radio)activity have been used including curie (1 Ci = 3.7

x 1010 disintegrations per second) and Becquerel ( 1 Bq = 1 disintegration per second).

**Actual focal-spot size:** The area on the anode target that is exposed to electrons from the tube current.

**Acute radiation syndrome :** Radiation sickness that occurs in humans after whole-body doses of 1Gy (100 rad) or more of ionising radiation delivered over a short time.

**Afterglow:** Phosphorescence in an intensifying screen.

**Air burst:** A nuclear weapon explosion that is high enough in the air to keep the fireball from touching the ground. Because the fireball does not reach the ground and does not pick up any surface material, the radioactivity in the fallout from an air burst is relatively insignificant compared with a surface burst.

**Air contrast:** Tecchnique of using air to outline soft tissue structures for radiographic contrast on film.

**Air gap technique:** A method of reducing scattered radiation to the film by separating the film and the object being examined by some distance. *e.g.,* the practice of moving the image receptor 10 to 15 cm from the patient so that fewer scattered X-rays interact with the image receptor, which enhances contrast of a radiograph.

**Ala:** Wing, wing like process or part.

**Alar:** Pertaining to an ala *e.g.* alar process of sacrum.

**ALARA:** Acronym for "As Low As Reasonably Achievable," means making every reasonable effort to maintain exposures to ionizing radiation as far below the dose limits as practical. This is a key principle in radiation protection and safety.

**Algia:** Suffix denoting pain *e.g.* arthralgia is pain in a joint.

**Alpha particle:** The particulate form of ionising radiation consisting of two protons and two neutrons. The nucleus of helium. Emitted from the nucleus of a radioactive atom.

**Alternating current (AC):** The oscillation of electricity in both directions in a conductor.

**Aluminum equivalent:** The thickness of aluminum affording the same attenuation, under specified conditions. Relates to radiation dose to the patients, the public, and occupationally exposed individuals.

**Amb prefix:** Meaning both *e.g.* ambilateral means affecting both sides.

**Amber filter:** A filter that transmits light with wavelengths longer than 550 nm, which is above the spectral response of blue-sensitive film.

**Ambient air:** The air that surrounds us.

**Ammeter:** An instrument that measures current.

**Ammonium thiosulfate:** Liquid fixing agent.

**Ampere (A):** The SI unit of electric charge. 1A=1C/s. The unit of measure used to describe the number of electrons or current flowing through the cathode filament.

**Amplification:** Magnifying ionisation impulses for measurement in radiation detection instruments.

**Amplitude:** The width of a waveform (maximum height of a wavelength crest).

**Anatomic:** Of pertaining to or dealing with body structure.

**Anechoic:** Not containing internal echoes (on ultrasound).

**Angiocardiography:** X-ray imaging of the heart and great vessels made visible by injection of a (radio-opaque) contrast solution.

**Angiogram:** An imaging study depicting blood vessels. In a conventional angiogram, a (radio-opaque) contrast is injected into the bloodstream and X-rays are taken to visualize the blood vessels. In other instances, CT or MRI can be used to create three-dimensional pictures of blood vessels.

**Angiography:** A medical imaging technique used to visualise the inside, or lumen, of blood vessels and organs of the body which are made visible by injection of a (radio-opaque) contrast solution.

**Angioma:** Tumour composed largely of blood vessels.

**Angstrom (An):** The unit of measure of wavelength.

**Anion:** A negatively charged ion, attracted to the anode.

**Anode:** The positively charged electrode of an X-ray tube which contains the target and from which X-rays are emitted. The target is usually composed on tungsten.Anodes may be either stationary or rotating.

**Ante:** Prefix denoting before (in time or place).

**Antegrade:** Moving in the direction considered normal.

**Anterior(ventral):** Toward the front; the opposite of posterior or dorsal.

**Anteroposterior (AP):** Directed or extending from front to back. A subject position where X-rays enter the anterior portion of the subject and exit posteriorly for image production.

**Anti:** Prefix signifying - against, counter or opposite.

**Aperture diaphragm:** A simple beam restricting device that attaches a lead lined metal diaphragm to the head of an X-ray tube.

**Aponeurosis:** Greek apo = from, and neuron = tendon (later applied to nerve cell and its fibres), fibrous or membranous sheet like tendon.

**Arteriography/ Arteriogram:** Radiography of arteries exposed to contrast media.

**Arthritis:** Inflammation of a joint or a state characterised by inflammation of joints.

**Arthrogram:** A radiographic examination of a joint after the introduction of contrast medium.

**Arthrosis:** Any joint or juncture uniting two bones.

**Artifact:** Any density or mark on a radiograph that is caused by something not belonging to the part of being X-rayed.

**Atom:** The smallest particle of an element that can enter into a chemical reaction.

**Atomic mass number:** The total number of protons and neutrons in the nucleus of an atom.

**Atomic mass unit (AMU):** The mass of a neutral atom of an element, expressed as one twelfth the mass of carbon, which has been arbitrarily assigned value of 12.

**Atomic number:** The total number of protons in the nucleus of an atom.

**Atomic weight:** The mass of an atom, expressed in atomic mass units. For example, the atomic number of helium-4 is 2, the atomic mass is 4, and the atomic weight is 4.00026.

**Attenuation:** A collective term for the processes (absorption and scattering) by which the energy of an X-ray beam is diminished in its passage through matter.

**Automatic brightness control (ABC):** A feature on a fluoroscope that allows the radiographer to select an image-brightness level that is subsequently maintained automatically by varying the kVp, the mAs or both.

**Automatic film processing:** A system incorporating processor, transporters, water, recirculation, replenishment and dryer sub systems which automatically processes film from developer through dried product.

**Autoradiography:** Production of an image by the photographic recording of natural radiation.

**Axial tomography:** Conventional tomography in which the plane of the image is parrallel with the long axis of the body and results in sagittal and coronal images.

**Axial:** Pertaining to axis of the body, part or thing, directed along axis or centre line.

**Backscatter radiation:** Refers to those scattered X-rays that go "back"toward the film.

**Balloon angioplasty:** An imaging procedure in which a balloon-tipped catheter is guided into an artery and advanced to a blockage or narrowing in a blood vessel. The balloon is then inflated to open the vessel, deflated and removed.

**Barium (Ba):** A metallic, alkaline, earth element; BA, atomic no. 56, atomic wt. 137.327.

**Barium enema:** The use of radiopaque barium contrast in a radiographic examination to image the colon, and define the anatomy of the large bowel and rectum.

**Barium sulfate($BaSO_4$):** A white insoluble radiopaque powder that is used as a contrast material to make certain body parts more visible in X-ray images. Radiopaque substances limit the penetration of X-rays and other forms of radiation.

**Barium swallow:** Also called an esophagram. An X-ray examination that assesses both the pharynx and esophagus in the upper gastrointestinal tract.

**Barrier:** Protective shields of radiation absorbing material. The thickness of the material depends on its absorbing qualities, the source of radiation and distance from source to protection area. A commonly used material is lead.

**Base:** Area that serves as a mechanical support for the active phosphor layer in a radiographic intensifying screen. Used to hold the emulsion layer of radiographic film.

**Beam angle:** The angle between the central axis of the radiation beam and the plane of the radiographic film.

**Beam axis:** The central line representing maximal ultrasound or X-ray intensity.

**Beam penetrability:** The ability of an X-ray beam to penetrate tissue.

**Beam restrictor:** A device that restricts the size of the X-ray field to only the anatomic structures of interest.

**Beam:** A unidirectional flow of electromagnetic radiation.

**Becquerel (Bq):** Special name for the SI units of radioactivity. One becquerel is equal to disintegration per second. 1 Bq = 0.027 × $10^{-9}$ Ci.

**Benign:** Not cancerous. May also be defined as non-malignant. Benign is also used to describe medical conditions that have a mild course.

**Beta particle (B particle):** Ionising radiation with characteristics of an electron, emitted from the nucleus of a radioactive atom.

**Bexxar®:** An iodine-131 agent used in radioimmuniotherapy to treat non-Hodgkin lymphoma.

**Bi:** Prefix signifying two or twice, *e.g.* bilateral is both sides.

**Bifid:** Latin bis = double, and findo = to split.

**Bifurcation:** Division into two branches; point of division.

**Bilateral:** Two sided; pertaining to two sides.

**Binding energy:** Binding force of an electron determined by the distance between the nucleus and the orbiting shells.

**Biological half-life:** The time required for one half of the amount of a substance, such as a radionuclide, to be expelled from the body by natural metabolic processes, not counting radioactive decay, once it has been taken in through inhalation, ingestion, or absorption.

**Biopsy:** Process of removing tissue from living patients for diagnostic examination or a specimen obtained by biopsy.

**Black marks:** This is an error made during processing caused by nail pressure to film,or possibly light or saliva leaks through the film packets.

**Black paper of film:** Goes around the front and back of film and helps protect the film from light and moisture if there is a leak in the outer wrapper.

**Blood brain barrier:** A specialized mechanism, not a structure, that inhibits the passage of certain materials from the blood into brain tissue and cerebrospinal fluid.

**Blurry film:** Little bit of exposure to the whole film, possible causes= incorrect filter, improper safe-light, incorrect bulb, or incorrect distance.

**Bolus:** A moistened mass of food that is swallowed from the oral cavity into the pharynx.

**Brachy:** Prefix meaning short, *e.g.* brachyfacial is a short broad face.

**Brachycephalic:** A head of short broad type.

**Brachytherapy:** A type of radiation therapy used to treat cancer, involving the placement of a radioactive material, either temporarily or permanently, directly inside the body.

**Bremsstrahlung X-ray :** An X-ray resulting from interaction of the projectile electron with a target nucleus, braking radiation.

**Bronchoscopy:** Visual inspection of the inside of the trachea and the bronchial passages of the lungs, using a rigid or flexible tube.

**Brown film/ image:** This is a processing error that is caused by insufficient fixing or washing.

**Bucky factor (B):** The ratio of incident radiation to transmitted radiation through a grid, the ratio of patient dose with and without a grid.

**Bucky (moving grid):** The movement is designed to blur the image of the lead strips of the grid in radiographs.

**Buffer:** Acetate added to the fixer to maintain a constant pH.

**Buffering agent:** An alkali compund in the developer that enhances the action of the developing agent by controlling the concentration of hydrogen ions.

**Cancer:** A tumor characterized by abnormally rapid cell division and the loss of specialized tissue characteristics. General term frequently used to indicate any of various types of malignant neoplasms.

**Carina:** A ridge at the tracheal bifurcation, formed by the last tracheal cartilage that runs antero-posteriorly between the orifices of the two main bronchi - from "carina" - the "v" shape of the bottom of a boat.

**C-arm:** A portable device for fluoroscopy. The opposite ends of the C-shaped support arm hold the image intensifier and the X-ray tube.

**Cassette:** A light-tight container for holding a radiographic film during exposure, a rigid holder that contains the film and the screens.

**Cassette-loaded spot film:** The conventional method of capturing images used with image-intensified fluoroscopes.

**Cata -prefix:** Signifying down lower, against, in accordance with, eg catabasis.

**Cathode ray tube (CRT):** An electron beam tube designed for two-dimensional display of signals.

**Cathode rays:** Electrode in the X-ray tube from which electrons are emitted. It consists of one or two filaments and focusing cup.

**Cathode:** A negative electrode.

**Caudal :** Nearer the tail (or where it would be). the kidneys are caudal to the diaphragm.

**Cele-suffix:** Signifying tumor or hernia *e.g.* cystocele a hernial protusion of the urinary bladder.

**Cell:** The structural and functional unit of an organism; the smallest structure capable of performing all the functions necessary for life.

**Cellulitis:** Inflammation of connective cellular tissue, especially of subcutaneous areas.

**Centesis:** Surgical puncture of a cavity, tapping.

**Centi:** Prefix denoting a hundred or hundredth part, used mainly in the metric system *e.g.* centimetre.

**Centigray:** 0.01 Gray (Gy). 1 of this is equal to 1 rad.

**Central axis X-ray beam:** An X-ray beam composed of X-rays traveling along the centre of the useful X-ray beam.

**Central Beam:** Central processing unit (CPU): the processing hardware in computers.

**Central Ray (Central Beam):** Refers to the X-rays in the center of the useful or primary beam.

**Cervical:** Pertaining to the neck or a neck like portion of an organ.

**Cervico:** Prefix indicating relation to neck or to cervix of any organ.

**Characteristic curve:** A curve expressing the relationship between radiation exposure to the film/screen combination and the resulting optical density.

**Characteristic radiation:** Discrete electromagnetic radiation is released as electrons move from higher (outer) to lower (inner) electron energy shells in an excited atom. Energy of the X-ray is unique to the element, therefore "characteristic". The energy of a characteristic X-ray is equal to the difference in binding energy of the two electron shells involved in the transition.

**Chemical energy:** The energy released by a chemical reaction.

**Chemical fog:** An artifact produced by chemical contamination of the developer.

**Chemotherapy:** Treatment of disease by means of chemical substances or drugs; usually used in reference to neoplastic (cancer) disease.

**Cholangiography:** Radiographic demonstration of bile ducts after they have been filled with radiopaque contrast medium.

**Cholecystectomy:** Is the surgical removal of the gallbladder.

**Cholecystitis:** Inflammation of the gallbladder.

**Cholecystography:** Radiographic demonstration of gallbladder following administration of substance that makes the organ radiopaque.

**Cholegraphy:** Radiologic examination of biliary tract by means of contrast medium.

**Cholelithiasis:** Being affected with cacluli in the bile duct.

**Choroid plexus:** Highly vascular secretary tissue found within the ventricular system in the brain, responsible for secreting cerebral spinal fluid.

**Chronic exposure:** Irradiation which is spread out over a period of years. Those who are occupationally exposed to radiation can suffer from chronic exposure.

**Chronic:** Continuing for a long time *e.g.* a chronic disease is one that is characterised by a protracted course, opposite of acute.

**Cicatrical:** Pertaining to or having character of a scar or cicatrix.

**Cine film:** The film used in cinefluorography.

**Cinefluorography:** The recording of fluoroscopic images on movie film.

**Clearing agent:** A chemical usually ammonium thiosulfate, added to the fixer to remove undeveloped silver bromide from the emulsion.

**Clearing time:** The time it takes for fixer to dissolve undeveloped silver halide, characterised by disappearance of milky diffusion on film after it is placed in fixer solution.

**Coherent scatter:** When an X-ray photon is scattered and no loss of energy occurs.

**Colitis:** Inflammation of the colon.

**Collimation:** The restriction of the size and shape of the X-ray beam in order to reduce patient exposure.

**Collimators:** An X-ray tube attachment for restricting the size and shape of the primary radiation beam. A variable collimator consists of two (and sometimes more) sets of independently adjustable lead shutters at right angles to each other, which provide a great variety of rectangular or square fields.

**Colo-prefix:** Denoting relation to colon *e.g.* colocentesis is a surgicalpuncture of the colon.

**Colon:** The first portion of the large intestine.

**Colonoscopy:** Visual examination of the inner surface of the colon by means of a lighted, flexible tubular instrument inserted into the colon through the rectum.

**Color Doppler:** Color doppler uses a computer to convert the Doppler measurements into an array of colors. This color visualization is combined with a standard ultrasound picture of a blood vessel to show the speed and direction of blood flow through the vessel.

**Colostomy:** Establishment of an artificial opening into the colon.

**Comets:** Artifacts produced on film that resemble comets. They are usually caused by rust particles adhering to film during development.

**Compton effect:** Attenuation process for X or gamma radiation. In this process the incident photon interacts with a free or loosely-bound electron, transferring a portion of the photon's energy to the electron termed as Compton electron.

**Compton scatter radiation:** The incident radiation has sufficient energy to dislodge a bound electron, but attacks a loosely bound electron, dislodges the electron and the remaining radiation energy proceeds in a different direction as scatter radiation. This kind of radiation is the main process responsible for the dose of radiation the patient receives during a radiographic procedure.

**Computed radiography (CR):** Radiographic technique that uses a photostimulable phosphor as the image receptor and an area beam.

**Computed tomography (CT) angiography:** Sometimes referred to as computerized axial tomography (CAT) scan is a method of examining blood vessels utilizing X-rays and injection of iodinated contrast medium.

**Cone:** A round/circular metal tube/shield attached to the X-ray tube housing or placed in front of the X-ray tube to limit the size of the X-ray beam to a predetermined size and shape.

**Cones and cylinders:** Modifications of the aperture diaphragm.

**Constant potential circuit:** A circuit which is arranged to supply a substantially constant voltage across an X-ray tube.

**Contra:** Prefix signifying against, in opposition *e.g.* contraindication.

**Contra lateral:** Taking place or originating in a corresponding part on the opposite side of the body.

**Contrast agent:** Also referred to as contrast or contrast medium. Any internally administered substance that has a different opacity from soft tissue on radiography or computed tomography.

**Contrast resolution:** The ability to distinguish between and to image similar tissues.

**Contrast:** In radiology, it is defined as the difference in density between light and dark areas on the processed film.

**Controlled area:** An area where personnel occupancy and activity are subject to control and supervision for the purpose of radiation protection.

**Conversion factor:** The ratio of the illumination intensity at the output phosphor to the radiation intensity incident on the input phosphor.

**Coolidge tube :** A type of vacuum tube in use today that allows X-ray intensity and energy to be separately and accurately selected.

**Cooling curve:** The graphic relaton between heat accumulation in an X-ray tube and the time it takes for the tube to cool.

**Cosmic radiation:** Radiation produced in outer space when heavy particles (nuclei of all known natural elements) bombard the earth.

**Cranial:** Pertaining to the cranium.

**Crossed grid:** A grid composed of two linear grids, one on top of the other, with the grid lines of one perpendicular to the grid lines of the other.

**Curie (Ci):** The former unit of radioactivity. Expressed as 1 Ci = 3.7 × $10^{1}$p disintegration per seconds = 3.7 × $10^{1}$p Bq.

**Curvilinear:** Having a curved configuration.

**Cystography/Cystogram:** Radiographic examination of urinary bladder after it has been filled with contrast medium.

**Cystoscopy:** Visual inspection of interior of urinary bladder by means of cytoscope.

**De novo:** From the beginning; a new.

**Densitometer:** An instrument used to measure film density which is degree of blackening of film by measuring the ratio of the light intensity incident on the film to the light intensity transmitted by the film.

**Density:** Film blackening (the amount of light transmitted through the film).

**Detail (definition):** Refers to the sharpness of structure lines or contour lines on the processed film.

**Detector:** A device that is sensitive to radiation and can produce a response signal suitable for measurement or analysis. A radiation detection instrument determines the amount of electrons passing through the cathode filament, an increase in he number of electrons available to travel from the cathode to the anode results in the production of an increased number of X-rays.

**Developer:** The chemical solution (alkaline) that converts the latent image on film to a visible image. It consistsof a developing agent (hydroquinone), an accelerator (sodium carbonate), a preservative (sodium sulfite) and a restrainer (potassium bromide) to prevent unexposed silver bromide crystals in film from blackening.

**Developing agent:** A chemical, usually phenidone, hydroquinone, or Metol, that reduces exposed silver ions to atomic silver.

**Developing:** The stage of processing during which the latent image is converted to a manifest image.

**Development:** The chemical reduction of the silver-halide ions to metallic silver of the exposed grains of the film emulsion.

**Diagnosis:** Art or act of determining character of a disease from existing symptoms; also conclusion reached.

**Diagnostic mammography:** Examination performed on patients with symptoms or elevated risk factors for breast cancer.

**Digital fluoroscopy (DF):** A digital X-ray imaging system that produces a series of dynamic images obtained with an area X-ray beam and an image intensifier.

**Direct current (DC):** The flow of electricity in only one direction in a conductor.

**Direct-exposure film:** Film used without intensifying screens.

**Dis -prefix :** Denoting abscence, reversal or seperation.

**Disc / disc space:** The space between the vertebrae, formed from a fibrous ring (the annulus) and a central "cushion" (nucleus pulposis).

**Discography:** Radiography of intervertebral discs exposed to contrast media.

**Distortion:** Unequal magnification of different portions of the same object, lack of (geometric) proportionality.

**Dose (radiation):** Radiation absorbed by a person's body. Several different terms describe radiation dose.

**Dose equivalent:** Means the product of the absorbed dose in tissue, quality factor, and all other necessary modifying factors at the location of interest. The unit of dose equivalent are the rem and the Sievert (Sv). 1 rem=0.01 Sv.

**Dose rate:** Absorbed dose (or dose equivalent) delivered per unit of time.

**Dosimeter:** A small portable instrument (such as a film badge, thermoluminescent dosimeter [TLD], or pocket dosimeter) for measuring and recording the total accumulated dose of ionizing radiation a person receives. In common use, a pencil size ionization chamber with a self-reading electrometer used for personnel monitoing.

**Dosimetry:** Assessment (by measurement or calculation) of radiation dose.

**Double contrast examination:** An examination of the colon that uses air and barium for contrast.

**Drying:** Film must be dried after washing. This is accomplished with controlled heat or time. A detergent rinse after washing will shorten drying time.

**Duplicating film:** A single-emulsion film that is exposed to ultraviolet light or blue light through the existing radiograph to produce a copy.

**Ec-prefix:** Meaning out or outside of.

**Eccentric:** Situated off center, not having same centre, opposed to concentric.

**Ecto-prefix:** Denoting without, on the outer side, external ego ectopic is out of normal position.

**Ectomy -suffix:** Denoting surgical removal *e.g.* cholecystectomy.

**Ectopic :** Greek ek = out, and topos = place, hence out of place.

**Eddy current:** A current opposing the magnetic field that induced it, creating a loss of transformer efficiency.

**Edema:** An excessive accumulation of fluid in the body tissues.

**Edge enhancement:** The accentuation of the interface between different tissues.

**Edison, Thomas:** Inventor Thomas Edison invented fluoroscopy and the fluoroscopic screen in 1896.

**Effective dose (E):** The sum over specified tissues of the products of the equivalent dose in a tissue and the weighting factor for the tissue.

**Electric current:** The flow of electrons.

**Electric field:** The lines of force exerted on charged ions in the tissues by the electrodes that cause charged particles to move from one pole to another.

**Electrical energy:** The work that can be done when an electron or an electronic charge moves through an electric potential.

**Electricity:** A form of energy created by the activity of electrons and other subatomic particles in motion.

**Electrode:** An electrical terminal or connector.

**Electromagnetic radiation:** Oscillating electric and magnetic fields that travel in a vacuum with the velocity of light. Includes X-rays, gamma rays, and some non-ionizing radiation.

**Electron binding energy:** The strength of attachment of an electron to the nucleus.

**Electron density:** The number of electrons per $cm^3$ in a material. Soft tissues including fat have very similar electron density; bone is nearly twice as high.

**Electron volt (eV):** The energy gained by an electron as it is accelerated through a potential difference of 1 volt.

**Electron:** An elementary particle with a negative electrical charge and a mass 1/1837 that of the proton. Electrons surround the nucleus of an atom because of the attraction between their negative charge and the positive charge of the nucleus. A stable atom will have as many electrons as it has protons. The number of electrons that orbit an atom determine its chemical properties.

**Electrostatic force:** Attraction between the positive nucleus and the negative electrons.

**em:** Prefix meaning in *e.g.* empyema is pus in a cavity.

**Emulsion:** The most important component of X-ray film. It is composed of silver halide crystals suspended in gelatin.

**Endo-prefix:** Meaning within; occupying an inward position *e.g.* endocarditis is inflammation of lining membrane of heart.

**Endoscopy:** Visual inspection of gastrointestinal tract with fiberoptic scope.

**Energy subtraction:** A technique that uses the two X-ray beams alternately to provide a subtraction image resulting from differences in photoelectric interaction.

**Envelope:** A glass tube surrounding the electrodes of an X-ray tube inside which a vacuum is maintained.

**Epi-prefix:** Meaning on, above, on the outside, over eg epigastric means situated above the stomach.

**Ex -prefix:** Denoting out, out of, or away from *e.g.* excavation is hollowing out.

**Exacerbation:** Increase in the severity of a disease or any of its symptoms.

**Excitation:** The addition of energy to a system by raising the energy of electrons with the use of X-rays.

**Exo-prefix:** Meaning outward or outside *e.g.* exogenous is growing from or on the outside of a part of body.

**Exposure (radiation):** A measure of ionization in air caused by X-rays or gamma rays only. The unit of exposure most often used is the roentgen.

**Exposure chart:** A chart on which is plotted one or more curves which indicate exposures for specified source or X-ray tube, product, film, film density and source to film distance for various product thicknesses.

**Exposure factors:** The factors that influence and determine the quantity and quality of X-radiation to which the patient is exposed.

**Exposure time:** kVp increased by 15 when kVp is increased by 15, exposure time must be cut in half. kVp is decreased by 15, when kVp is decreased by 15, exposure time must be doubled.

**Extra -prefix:** Meaning on outside, beyond, in addition *e.g.* extragastric is situated or occuring outside the stomach.

**Extrapolation:** The estimation of a value beyond the range of known values.

**Field of view (FOV):** The image matrix size provided by digital X-ray imaging systems.

**Filament:** The part of the cathode that emits electrons, resulting in a tube current.

**Film badge:** A pack of photographic film used for approximate measurement of radiation exposure to radiation workers. It is the most widely used and most economical type of personnel radiation monitor.

**Film contrast:** The contribution to the overall radiographic contrast from the intensifying screen-film processing system visualised in a processed radiograph. Film contrast usually increases the subject contrast (i.e., gamma is greater that one) as the system converts the X-ray intensity variations emergent from the subject into visible images.

**Film emulsion:** Coating on film base.

**Film fog:** All or part of the radiograph is darkened by sources other than the primary beam.

**Film packet:** Contents waterproof outer layer, black paper, film, lead foil.

**Film sensitivity:** Determines how much radiation for what period of time(mAs) is needed to produce an image on the film.

**Film Speed:** Film speed change problem formula with each change in speed, the exposure time needed halves, with each decrease in speed, the exposure time needed doubles.

**Film Speed:** A relative exposure number needed to produce a density of 1/0 above gross fog-used for screen type, dental and medical X-ray films.

**Film:** To capture and make a permanent image, has an outer protective coating on front and back.

**Filter/Filtration:** The removal of low-energy X-rays from the useful beam with aluminum, copper or another metal. It results in increased beam quality and reduced patient dose.

**First-generation computed tomographic scanner:** A finely collimated X-ray beam, single-detector assembly that translates across the patient and rotates between successive translations.

**Fixation:** The removal of undeveloped silver halide grains after development of the film to prevent slow darkening, which would otherwise occur as the silver ions are gradually, naturally reduced over time.

**Fixer:** A chemical solution (acidic) which removes the unexposed and underdeveloped silver halide crystals from the film so it will not discolor or darken with age or exposure to light. Also hardens the gelatin containing the black metallic silver so film may be dried and resist damage from abrasions.

**Fixing:** The stage of processing during which the silver halide not exposed to radiation is dissolved and removed from the emulsion.

**Fluorescence:** The emission of visible light only during stimulation.

**Fluorescent screen:** The cycle in a television-picture tube when the electron beam creates the television optical signal and then immediately fades.

**Fluoroscopy:** An imaging modality that provides a continuous image of the motion of internal structures while the X-ray tube is energised. It is a type of real-time imaging.

**Focal Spot:** A small area on the target of the anode toward which the electrons from the focusing cup of the cathode are directed. X-radiation originates from here.

**Focused grid:** A radiographic grid constructed so that the grid strips converge on an imaginary line.

**Focusing cup:** A metal shroud surrounding the filament.

**Fog or Fogging:** A cloudy appearance of the finished radiograph caused by several factors such as old or contaminated processing solutions, exposure to chemical fumes, faulty darkroom safelight, or scatter radiation.

**Fractionated exposure:** Exposure to radiation that occurs in several small acute exposures, rather than continuously as in a chronic exposure.

**Fundamental particles:** The three primary constituents of an atom electrons, photons, and neutrons.

**Gamma rays:** High-energy electromagnetic radiation emitted by certain radionuclides when their nuclei transition from a higher to a lower energy state. These rays have high energy and a short wave-length. All gamma rays emitted from a given isotope have the same energy, a characteristic that enables scientists to identify which gamma emitters are present in a sample. Gamma rays penetrate tissue farther than do beta or alpha particles but leave a lower concentration of ions in their path to potentially cause cell damage. Gamma rays are very similar to X-rays.

**Gantry:** The portion of the computed tomographic or magnetic resonance imaging system that accommodates the patient and source or the detector assemblies.

**Geiger-Muller counter:** Radiation-detection and radiation-measuring instrument that detects individual ionisations. It is the primary radiation survey instrument for nuclear medicine facilities. Geiger counters are the most commonly used portable radiation detection instruments.

**Gelatin:** The part of the emulsion that provides mechanical support for the silver halide crystals by holding them uniformly dispersed in place.

**Genetic effects:** Hereditary effects (mutations) that can be passed on through reproduction because of changes in sperm or ova.

**Geometric unsharpness:** Unsharpness of the recording image due to the combined optical effect of finite size of the radiation source and geometric separation of the anatomic area of interest from the image receptor and the collimator.

**Gonad Shielding:** Devices used during radiographic procedures to protect the reproductive organs from exposure to the useful X-ray beams.

**Gonadal dose:** The exposure to the reproductive organs. Gradient The slope of the tangent at any point on the characteristic curve.

**Gravel:** Deposit of small, stone like concretions in kidneys and urinary bladder: calculi.

**Gray (Gy):** The new international system (SI) unit of radiation dose, expressed as absorbed energy per unit mass of tissue. The SI unit "Gray" has replaced the older "rad" designation. (1 Gy = 1 joule/ kilogram = 100 rad). Gray can be used for any type of radiation (e.g., alpha, beta, neutron, gamma), but it does not describe the biological effects of different radiations. Biological effects of radiation are measured in units of "Sievert" (or the older designation "rem"). Sievert is calculated as follows: Gray multiplied by the "radiation weighting factor" (also known "quality factor") associated with a specific type of radiation.

**Gray scale:** An image display in which intensity is recorded as variations in brightness.

**Grid cut-off:** The absence of optical density on a radiograph because of unintended X-ray absorption in a grid.

**Grid frequency:** The number of grid lines per inch or centimeter.

**Grid lines:** A series of sections of radiopaque material.

**Grid ratio:** The ratio of grid height to grid strip separation.

**Grid:** A device used to reduce scatter radiation in the remnant X-ray beam. Constructed of alternating strips of lead and a radio-transparent medium (such as aluminum, wood, or plastic) which are oriented in such a way that most of the primary radiation: will pass through the grid between the strips while most of the scattered radiation will intersect the lead strips and be absorbed.

**Grid-controlled tube:** An X-ray tubes designed to be turned on and off very rapidly for situations requiring multiple exposures at precise exposure times.

**Ground glass:** Any extended, finely granular pattern of pulmonary opacity within which normal anatomic details are partially (not completely) obscured. Compare with consolidation, in which the underlying anatomic details are completely obscured.

**Half-life:** The time any substance takes to decay by half of its original amount.

**Hard copy:** A permanent image on film or paper, as opposed to an image on a cathode ray tube, disk, or magnetic tape.

**Hard X-ray:** An X-ray that has high penetrability and therefore is of high quality.

**Hardener:** A chemical, usually potassium glutaraldehyde in the fixer, that is used to stiffen and shrink the emulsion.

**Hardware:** The visible parts of the computer.

**Heel effect:** A consequence of the angle of the target of the tube which results in greater radiation intensities on the cathode side as compared to the anode side of the radiation field.

**Hem-, haem-, hemo -prefix:** Denoting blood or relation to blood: as hematuria, presence of blood in urine.

**Hemangioma:** Tumor consisting of newly formed blood vessels.

**Hematogenous:** Spread by means of the blood stream.

**Hemi-prefix:** Signifying one half; pertaining to or affecting one side of body; as hemiplegia, paralysis of one side of body.

**Hertz (Hz):** The unit of frequency; the number of cycles or oscillations each second of a simple harmonic motion.

**High contrast:** A term describing an image with many very dark areas and very light areas and few shades of gray.

**High-contrast resolution:** The ability to image small objects having high subject contrast; spatial resolution.

**High-voltage generator:** One of three principal parts of an X-ray imaging system; it is always close to the X-ray tube.

**Hit:** Radiation interaction with the target.

**Homeo-prefix:** Meaning like, similar; as homeomorphous, of similar structure and form.

**Horizontal(transverse, axial) plane:** A directional plane that divides the body, organ, or appendage into superior and inferior or proximal and distal portions.

**horsepower (hp):** The British unit of power.

**Hot spot:** Any place where the level of radioactive contamination is considerably greater than the area around it.

**Hounds field unit (HU):** The scale of computed tomographic numbers used to judge the nature of tissue.

**Hydroquinone:** The principal compound used in the chemical composition of film developers.

**Hysterography:** Radiographic examination of uterus after injection of contrast medium; uterography.

**Hystero-prefix:** Denoting relation to uterus; as hysterectomy, surgical removal of uterus.

**Hysterosalpingography:** Radiographic examination of uterus and oviducts after injection of contrast medium; uterosalpingography.

**-iasis suffix:** Denoting morbid or diseased condition; as elephantiasis, nephrolithiasis, dracontiasis.

**Iatrogenic:** Resulting from the activity of physicians.

**Idio-:** Prefix combining form denoting self-produced; as idiopathic, self-originated, of unknown cause.

**Ileo-prefix:** Denoting some relation to ileum; as ileocolic, ileocecal, ileotomy.

**im- , in- prefixes:** Meaning in, within, or into, as in immersion, injection; also, not, non-, un-, as in imbalance, inactive, incurable.

**Image detail:** The sharpness of small structures on the radiograph.

**Image intensifier:** An electronic vacuum tube that amplifies a fluoroscopic image to reduce patient dose.

**Indolent:** Causing little or no pain; slow to heal.

**Infarction:** Death of tissue because of interruption of the normal blood supply.

**Infra-prefix:** Meaning below; as infraorbital, situated below orbit.

**Inherent filter:** Filter in the X-ray tube and its housing such as the glass envelope (window) through which the X-ray beam passes.

**Initiation time:** The time required to start an exposure.

**Insidious:** Developing in a slow or not apparent manner; more dangerous than seems evident, as in an insidious disease.

**Installation:** The location where one or more reportable sources of radiation are processed (located).

**Insulator:** A material that inhibits the flow of electrons in a conductor or in heat transfer.

**Intensifying screen:** A device that transfers X-ray energy into visible light; the visible light in turn , which increase the brightness of the image produced by the action of X-rays upon a phosphor. With its use less radiation is required to expose screen film, and patient is exposed to less radiation.

**Intensity:** The total energy passing through a unit area per unit time.

**Inter- prefix:** Signifying between; as interlobar, situated between two lobes.

**Interface:** The boundary between the shadows of two juxtaposed structures or tissues of different texture or opacity.

**Internal exposure:** Exposure to radioactive material taken into the body.

**Interstitial:** Referring to the area between cells.

**Intra-prefix:** Meaning within or into; as intralobar, within a lobe, and intravenous, injected into a vein.

**Inverse square law:** Law stating that the intensity of the radiation at a location is inversely proportional to the square of its distance from the source of radiation.

***In-vivo*:** Occurring within the body, in the living cell.

**Iodine:** A nonmetallic solid element. There are both radioactive and non-radioactive isotopes of iodine. Radioactive isotopes of iodine are widely used in medical applications. Radioactive iodine is a fission product and is the largest contributor to people's radiation dose after an accident at a nuclear reactor.

**Ion chamber:** An instrument that detects and measures the radiation intensity in areas outside of protective barriers.

**Ion pair:** Two oppositely charged particles.

**Ion:** An atom or molecule which has one or more of its surrounding electrons separated from it and therefore carries a positive electric charge, or a free electron carrying a negative electrical charge.

**Ionic bonds:** A bonding that occurs because of an electrostatic force between ions.

**Ionisation chamber:** A device for measuring exposure by collecting the electrical charge carried by the ions produced in a finite air volume by the incident radiation.

**Ionising radiation:** Radiation capable of ionisation. High-energy electromagnetic radiation that produces ions as it passes through matter e.g. X-rays, gamma rays, and some energies of ultraviolet radiation. On average, 33 eV is required to ionise a water molecule.

**Ionization:** The production of ions, the process of converting an atom into an ion, deals only with energy to overcome the electrostatic force that binds the electron to the nucleus, resulting in the formation of a positive atom and a dislodged negative electron.

**Ionized:** Referring to an atom that has an extra electron or has had an electron removed.

**Irradiated:** Referring to matter that intercepts radiation and absorbs part or all of it; exposed.

**Irradiation:** Exposure to radiation.

**Isobars:** Atoms having the same number of nucleons but different numbers of protons and neutrons.

**Isomers:** Atoms having the same number of protons and neutrons but a different nuclear energy state.

**Isotones:** Atoms having the same number of neutrons.

**Isotope:** A nuclide of an element having the same number of protons but a different number of neutrons.

**Isotopic tracer:** The isotopic or non-natural mixture of isotopes of an element which may be incorporated into a sample to make observation of the course of that element, alone or in combination, through a chemical, biological or physical process.

**-itis suffix:** Signifying inflammation of specified part; as arthritis, appendicitis, bronchitis.

**kilo electron volt(keV):** The kinetic energy gained by an electron as a result of being accelerated through a potential difference of 1,000 volts (equal to 1,000 eV or 1 keV).

**Kilovolt peak (kVp):** A unit of maximum or crest value of electrical potential difference between the anode and cathode of an X-ray tube; determines the penetrating ability of X-rays and revers to the "quality" of X-rays.

**Kilo-voltage(kV):** Can be adjusted according to the individual diagnostic needs of the patient. The use of 85 to 100 kV produces more penetrating X-rays with greater energy and shorter wavelengths, 65 to 70 kV produces less penetrating dental X-rays with less energy and longer wavelengths. A higher kV should be used when the examined area is dense or thick. 1 likovolt is = 1000 volts.

**Kinetic energy:** The energy of motion.

**kVp:** The maximum of peak voltage that is used during an X-ray exposure. Low kVp=short scale=high contrast; High kVp=long scale=low contrast.

**Kymography:** Radiographic recording of involuntary movements of such viscera as heart, stomach, and diaphragm, and motion, as in blood vessels.

**Latent Image:** Invisible image formed on the exposed film which becomes visible after film undergoes chemical processing.

**Latent period:** The amount of time that lapses between exposure to ionizing radiation and the appearance of observable clinical signs.

**Lead (Pb):** A heavy metal. Several isotopes of lead, such as Pb-210 which emits beta particles, are in the uranium decay chain.

**Lead apron:** A flexible lead shield used to protect the patients reproductive and blood forming tissues from scatter radiation.

**Leakage radiation:** Means all radiation coming from within the X-ray tube housing except the useful beam.

**Lethal dose (50/30):** The dose of radiation expected to cause death within 30 days to 50% of those exposed without medical treatment. The generally accepted dose is about 400 rem received over a short period of time.

**Leukemia:** A blood disease which is characterized by overproduction of white blood cells. It may result from overexposure of the bone marrow to radiation.

**Linear opacity:** A shadow resembling a line; an elongated opacity of uniform width, qualified with regard to length,width, orientation, and anatomic location.

**Long scale contrast films:** Low contrast films, many gray tones, 90 to 100 kVp, early detection of bone loss and incipient decay.

**Long scale of contrast :** A term describing an image with many densities, or many shades of gray; it results from the use of a higher kilo-voltage range; Longer wavelengths=less penetrating and more likely to be absorbed by matter.

**Low contrast:** A term describing an image with many shades of gray and few areas of black and white.

**Low kilovoltage peak settings (65-70 kVp) :** Creates a high contrast film many black and white areas, few shades of gray.

**Lucency:** The ability to transmit light, and thus the ability to transmit X-radiation.

**Macro-prefix:** Signifying excessive development, especially elongation; as macrocephalic, an unusually large head; also, morbid enlargement; as macrencephaly, hypertrophy or enlargement of the brain; opposed to micro.

**Magnetic dipole:** Current flowing in an infinitesimally small loop.

**Magnification:** The ratio of image size to object size. The image may be larger than, smaller than, or equal to the object; so magnification can be greater than, equal to, or less than 1.

**Mal-prefix:** Meaning ill, bad, badly; as malalignment, malfunction. maldevelopment.

**Mammographer:** A radiologic technologist specialising in breast X-ray studies.

**Mammography:** Radiographic examination of the breast also called mastography.

**mAs (milliampere seconds):** mAs is an acronym for milliampere-seconds. A combination unit which is the product of the tube current (expressed in mA) and the exposure time (expressed in seconds). The total output of an X-ray tube is directly proportional to the mAs (or either of its components).

**Mask image:** The image obtained from mask mode.

**Masking:** The act of ensuring that no extraneous light from the viewbox enters the viewer's eyes.

**Mass :** A pulmonary or pleural lesion represented in a radiograph by a discrete opacity 30 mm or greater in diameter, explicitly shown or presumed to be extended in all three dimensions. Should be qualified with regard to opacity (especially presence of calcification), homogeneity, border characteristics, location, and number.

**Mass density:** The quantity of matter per unit volume.

**Masto-prefix:** Denoting relation to breast, as in mastocarcinoma, mastitis.

**Matter:** Anything that occupies space and has form or shape.

**Maximum permissible dose (MPD):** The dose of radiation that would be expected to produce no significant radiation effects.

**Mechanical energy:** The ability of an object to do work.

**Megalo -prefix:** Meaning large, great, abnormal enlargement; as megalo-esophagus, megalakria, acromegaly.

**Meta -prefix:** Signifying change or transfer, as in metabolism, metabasis: along with, after, or next, as in metatarsus.

**Metastasis:** Transfer of a disease from one organ or region to another, as a malignant tumor spreading from initial location to secondary locations in body.

**Metro-prefix:** Denoting relation to uterus, as in metrocarcinoma metrins.

**Microwave:** A short-wavelength radiofrequency.

**Midsagittal plane:** A plane that divides the body into equal right and left halves; also called the median plane or midplane.

**Milliampere (mA):** The electron current towing across the X-ray tube from the cathode to the anode.

**Milliampere-seconds (mAs):** Milliampere (mA) multiplied by the time during which the beam strikes an object (measured in seconds) is mAs and is a measure of the "quality" of X-rays.

**Molecule:** A combination of two or more atoms that are chemically bonded. A molecule is the smallest unit of a compound that can exist by itself and retain all of its chemical properties.

**Molybdenum:** A target material for X-ray tubes that is used in mammography.

**Monitoring:** Determining the amount of ionizing radiation or radioactive contamination present.

**Mono- prefix:** Meaning one, single, alone; as monoplegia, paralysis affecting but one part of body.

**Moving grid:** A grid that moves while the X-ray exposure is being made.

**MPD (Maximum Permissible Dose):** Maximum dose of radiation not expected to produce negative effects.

**Mutation:** A transformation of the gene which may be induced by radiation and may alter characteristics of the offspring.

**Myocardial infarction:** An area of necrotic tissue in the myocardium that is filled in by scar (connective) tissue.

**Myo -prefix:** Signifying relation to a muscle or muscles; as myocarditis, myositis.

**Neoplastic:** Pertaining to the pathologic process resulting in the formation and growth of an abnormal mass of tissue.

**Neutron:** A small atomic particle possessing no electrical charge, typically found within an atom's nucleus. Neutrons are, as the name implies, neutral in their charge. That is, they have neither a positive nor a negative charge. A neutron has about the same mass as a proton.

**Nuclear energy:** The heat energy produced by the process of nuclear fission within a nuclear reactor or by radioactive decay.

**Nuclear reactor:** A device in which a controlled, self-sustaining nuclear chain reaction can be maintained with the use of cooling to remove generated heat.

**Nuclear tracers:** Radioisotopes that give doctors the ability to "look" inside the body and observe soft tissues and organs, in a manner similar to the way X-rays provide images of bones. A radioactive tracer is chemically attached to a compound that will concentrate naturally in an organ or tissue so that an image can be taken.

**Nucleon:** A proton or aneutron; a constituent of the nucleus of an atom.

**Nucleus:** The central part of an atom that contains protons and neutrons. The nucleus is the heaviest part of the atom.

**Nuclide:** A general term applicable to all atomic forms of an element. Nuclides are characterized by the number of protons and neutrons in the nucleus, as well as by the amount of energy contained within the atom.

**Off-focus radiation:** Electrons that bounce off the focal spot and land on other areas of the target.

**One rad:** The dose corresponding to the absorption of 100 ergs per gram. 0.01= One rad.

**Opacity:** The capacity to attenuate an X-ray beam; the degree of attenuation of the X-ray beam, usually expressed in terms of the attenuation of one absorber to another. In a radiograph, an opacity is a circumscribed area that appears nearly white (i.e., denser) than its surroundings. Use of the term opacity does not imply location; opacity may be parenchymal, pleural, within the chest wall, or external to the patient.

**Penetrating radiation:** Radiation that can penetrate the skin and reach internal organs and tissues. Photons (gamma rays and X-rays), neutrons and protons are penetrating radiations. However, alpha particles and all but extremely high-energy beta particles are not considered penetrating radiation.

**Penumbra:** Fuzzy border of an object as imaged radiographically.

**Personal dosimeters:** Devices designed to be worn or carried by an individual for the purpose of determining the dose equivalent received for example:

Film badge, pocket chamber, pocket dosimeter, ring badges, thermoluminescent (TLD) badges, etc.

**Photon:** In physics, a corpuscle of energy or particle, a quantum of light energy.

**Pixel (picture element):** Tiny square making up the image matric, represent voxel.

**Primary barrier:** Barrier sufficient to attenuate the useful beam to the required degree.

**Primary radiation or X-ray beam:** That part of the radiation which passes through the window, aperture, cone, or other collimating device of the tube housing. Also called useful beam.

**Primary radiation:** The penetrating X-ray beam that is produced at the target (anode).

**Protective barrier:** Barrier of attenuating materials used to reduce radiation exposure.

**Protective coat /layer:** Protects the emulsion from damage.

**Proton:** A small atomic particle, typically found within an atom's nucleus, that possesses a positive electrical charge. Even though protons and neutrons are about 2,000 times heavier than electrons, they are tiny. The number of protons is unique for each chemical element.

**Quality factor (Q):** The linear energy transfer dependent factor by which absorbed doses arre multiplied to obtain a quantity that expresses, on common scale for all ionizing radiations, the effectiveness of the absorbed dose.

**Quality:** A term used to describe the penetrating power of X-rays and is related to the energies of the photons in the useful or primary X-ray beam.

**Quantity:** This of the X-ray beam refers to the number of X-rays produced in the X-ray machine

**Rad (radiation absorbed dose):** A basic unit of absorbed radiation dose. It is a measure of the amount of energy absorbed by the body. The rad is the traditional unit of absorbed dose. It is being replaced by the unit gray (Gy), which is equivalent to 100 rad. One rad equals the dose delivered to an object of 100 ergs of energy per gram of material.

**Radiation protection /radiological protection:** Is the science of protecting people and the environment from the harmful effects of ionizing radiation, which includes both particle radiation and high energy electromagnetic radiation. radiation that is deflected from its path as it strikes matter.

**Radiation:** Energy that is carried in the form of rays or waves or particles.

**Radioactive contamination:** The deposition of unwanted radioactive material on the surfaces of structures, areas, objects, or people. It can be airborne, external, or internal. Radioactive decay: the spontaneous disintegration of the nucleus of an atom.

**Radioactive material:** Material that contains unstable (radioactive) atoms that give off radiation as they decay.

**Radioactivity:** The process by which certain unstable atoms or elements undergo spontaneous disintegration, or decay, in an effort to attain a more balanced nuclear state.

**Radioassay:** A test to determine the amounts of radioactive materials through the detection of ionizing radiation. Radioassays will detecttransuranic nuclides, uranium, fission and activation products, naturally occurring radioactive material, and medical isotopes.

**Radiogenic:** Health effects caused by exposure to ionizing radiation.

**Radiography:** 1) Medical: the use of radiant energy (such as X-rays and gamma rays) to image body systems; 2) industrial: the use of radioactive sources to photograph internal structures, such as turbine blades in jet engines. A sealed radiation source, usually iridium-192 (Ir-192) or cobalt-60 (Co-60), beams gamma rays at the object to be checked. Gamma rays passing through flaws in the metal or incomplete welds strike special photographic film (radiographic film) on the opposite side.

**Radiography:** Utilizing ionizing radiation, this technique involves making shadow images on photographic emulsions. The image is the result of differences in attenuation of the radiation as it passes through the object in its path.

**Radioisotope (radioactive isotope):** Isotopes of an element that have an unstable nucleus.

**Radiolucent:** The portion of an image that is dark or black; this structure readily permits the passage of the X-ray beam and allows more X-rays to reach the receptor.

**Radioluminescence:** The luminescence produced by particles emitted during radioactive decay.

**Radionuclide:** An unstable and therefore radioactive form of a nuclide.

**Radiopaque:** The portion of an image that is light or white, this structure is one that resists the passage of the X-ray beam and limits the amount of X-rays that reach the receptor.

**Rads:** The dose equivalent in rems is equal to the absorbed dose in rads multiplied by the quality factor (1 rem - 0.01 Sievert).

**Relative biological effectiveness (RBE):** A factor used in radiobiology to compare the biological effectiveness of absorbed radiation doses (that is rad) due to different types of ionizing radiation, more specifically. It is the experimentally determined ratio of an absorbed dose of a reference radiation required to produce an identical biological effect in a particular experimental organism or tissue.

**Relative risk:** The ratio between the risk for disease in an irradiated population to the risk in an unexposed population. A relative risk of 1.1 indicates a 10% increase in cancer from radiation, compared with the "normal" incidence.

**Rem (roentgen equivalent, man):** A unit of equivalent dose. Not all radiation has the same biological effect, even for the same amount of absorbed dose. Rem relates the absorbed dose in human tissue to the effective biological damage of the radiation. It is determined by multiplying the number of rads by the quality factor, a number reflecting the potential damage caused by the particular type of radiation. The rem is the traditional unit of equivalent dose, but it is being replaced by the sievert (Sv), which is equal to 100 rem. Repeats/retakes: additional radiographs taken because of technical or mechanical error. These lead to increased radiation exposure for the patient and the radiation worker and should be avoided.

**Resolution:** The process or capability of distinguishing closely adjacent optical images.

**Risk assessment:** An evaluation of the risk to human health or the environment by hazards. Risk assessments can look at either existing hazards or potential hazards.

**Risk:** The probability of injury, disease, or death under specific circumstances and time periods. Risk can be expressed as a value that ranges from 0% (no injury or harm will occur) to 100% (harm or injury will definitely occur).

**Roentgen (R):** A unit of exposure to X-rays or gamma rays. One roentgen is the amount of gamma or X-rays needed to produce ionscarrying 1 electrostatic unit of electrical charge in 1 cubic centimeter of dry air under standard conditions.

**Roentgen equivalent man (rem):** Radiation unit of measurement.

**Safelight:** An incandescent lamp with a color filter that provides sufficient illumination in the darkroom while ensuring that the film remains unexposed.

**Sagittal plane:** Any anterior-posterior plane parallel to the long axis of the body.

**Scale of contrast:** The range of useful densities seen on a dental image.

**Scanned projection radiography (SPR):** Generalized method of making a digital radiograph; used in computed tomography for precision localisation.

**Scattered radiation:** Means radiation that during passage through matter, has been deviated in direction. It usually has also been modified by a decrease in energy.

**Scintillation detector:** An instrument used in the detector arrays of many computed tomographic scanners.

**Sclera- prefix:** Meaning hard, indurated, fibrous: also denotes relation to sclera of eye.

**Scoliosis:** Abnormal lateral curvature of the spinal column.

**Screen lag:** The phosphorescence in an intensifying screen.

**Screen speed:** A relative number used to identify the efficiency of conversion of X-rays into usable light. Second (s) the standard unit of time.

**Screen unsharpness:** The image unsharpness due to the size of the fluorescent crystals comprising the screens, the thickness of the screens, and/or the closeness of contact between the film and the screens.

**Screen-film:** Film made with thin emulsions (single- or double-sided) that is sensitive to either the blue or green light of fluorescent screens. Film should be matched to screen emissions.

**Secondary barrier:** Barrier sufficient to attenuate stray radiation to the required degree.

**Secondary coil:** The coil in which the induced current in an electromagnet flows.

**Secondary electron:** The ejected electron from the outer shell of an atom.

**Secondary or stray radiation:** Mean radiation not serving any useful purpose. It includes leakage and scattered radiation.

**Secondary protective barrier:** Barriers designed to shield areas from secondary radiation.

**Secondary radiation:** X-radiation created when the primary beam interacts with a matter.

**Second-generation computed tomographic scanner:** A unit that incorporates the natural extension of the single-detector to a multiple-detector assembly intercepting a fan-shaped rather than a pencil-shaped X-ray beam.

**Section thickness:** The thickness of tissue that will not be blurred by tomography. The section thickness decreases as tomographic angle increases.

**Selectivity:** The ratio of primary radiation to scattered radiation transmitted through grid.

**Self-induction:** The magnetic field produced in a coil of wire that opposes the alternating current being conducted.

**Self-rectified circuit:** The X-ray tube itself serves as a rectifier where only the positive portion of the AC cycle is used; therefore, it is a type of half-wave rectified circuit.

**Semi-prefix meaning partly :** Half or approximately half; as semiflexion, semiprone, semicoma.

**Shells:** The orbital energy levels surrounding the nucleus of an atom.

**Shield/Shielding:** Material which is interposed between a radiation source and an irradiated site for the purpose of minimizing the radiation hazard (used to prevent or reduce the passage of radiation). Usually made of lead which is dense and absorbs radiation easily. Used to protect the reproductive organs, testes or ovaries, from the X-ray beam during an examination.

**Sialography:** Radiographic examination of a salivary gland or duct after injection of radiopaque contrast medium.

**Sievert (Sv):** A unit used to derive a quantity called dose equivalent. This relates the absorbed dose in human tissue to the effective biological damage of the radiation. Not all radiation has the same biological effect, even for the same amount of absorbed dose. Dose equivalent is often expressed as millionths of a sievert, or micro-sieverts (μSv). One sievert is equivalent to 100 rem=1 Jkg.

**Silhouette sign:** The effacement of an anatomic soft tissue border by consolidation of the adjacent lung or accumulation of fluid in the contiguous pleural space. This is a sign of conformity, and, hence, of the probable adjacency of a pathologic opacity to a known structure. The silhouette sign is useful for detecting and localizing consolidation along the axis of the X-ray beam.

**Silver Bromide:** The material that makes up 98% of the silver halide crystals in a typical emulsion.

**Silver halide crystals:** The active ingredient of the radiographic emulsion. It is instrumental in creating a latent image on the radiograph.

**Silver iodide:** 5% of the silver halide crystals. Silver nitrate + potassium iodide.

**Silver iodide:** The material that makes up 2% of the silver halide crystals in a typical emulsion.

**Sine wave:** The variation of movement of photons in electrical and magnetic fields.

**Sinistrad:** Directed toward left; opposite of dextrad.

**Sinistro-prefix:** Meaning left, as in sinistrocardia, sinistrocerebral.

**Sinusoidal:** Simple motion; a sine wave.

**Skiagram/Skiagraph:** Old term for radiograph or roentgenogram.

**Sludge:** Deposits on the film resulting from dirty or warped rollers, causing emulsion pick-off and gelatin buildup.

**Sodium carbonate:** An alkali compound contained in the developer.

**Sodium hydroxide:** An alkali compound contained in the developer.

**Sodium sulfite:** The preservative added to the developer that keeps it clear.

**Soft copy:** The output on a display screen.

**Soft tissue radiograph:** Radiography in which only muscle and fat structures are imaged.

**Soft X-ray:** An X-ray that has low penetrability and therefore is of low quality.

**Software:** The computer programs that tell the hardware what to do and how to store data.

**Solution:** A suspension of particles or molecules in a fluid.

**Solvent:** A liquid into which various solids and powders can be dissolved.

**Somatic cells:** All the cells of the body except the oogonium and spermatogonium.

**Somatic effects:** Effects of radiation that are limited to the exposed person, as distinguished from genetic effects, which may also affect subsequent generations. See also teratogenic effects.

**Somatic:** Retaining to the body tissue other than reproductive cellsor nonvisceral parts of the body.

**Source-to-Image Distance (SID):** The distance measured along the central ray from the center of the front surface of the source X-ray focal spot to the surface of the irradiated object or patient.

**Source-to-skin distance (SSD):** The distance from the patient's skin to the fluoroscopic tube.

**Spatial frequency:** The measure of resolution; usually expressed in line pairs per millimeter (lp/mm).

**Spatial resolution:** The ability to image small objects that have high subject contrast.

**Spectrum:** The population of photons, usually plotted as intensity versus energy, see X-ray spectra.

**Sphygmomanometer:** A manometer (pressure transducer) used to measure the blood pressure.

**Spiral/helical:** The term given to computed tomography because it is the apparent motion of the X-ray tube during the scan.

**Spiral pitch ratio:** The relationship between the patient couch movement and X-ray beam collimation.

**Spot film:** Static image in small-format image receptor taken during fluoroscopy.

**Square law:** The principle stating that one can compensate for a change in the source-to-object distance by changing the mAs by the factor source to image distance (SID) squared.

**Stable nucleus:** The nucleus of an atom in which the forces among its particles are balanced.

**Staging:** Determination of the amount of spread of a neoplasm, necessary to select appropriate therapy and to predict the future course of a disease.

**Stationary anode:** An X-ray tube design in which the anode is a single immobile structure.

**Step wedge:** A filter used when radiographing a body part, such as the foot, that varies in thickness from one end to the other.

**Step-down transformer:** A transformer in which the voltage is decreased from the primary side to the secondary side.

**Stepping:** A computer-controlled capability on a patient table that allows imaging from the abdomen to the feet after a single injection of contrast media.

**Step-up transformer:** A transformer in which the voltage is increased from the primary side to the secondary side.

**Stereoradiography:** The practice of making two radiographs of the same object and viewing through a device which allows each eye to view a different radiograph.

**Stochastic effects:** The probability or frequency of the biologic response to radiation as a function of radiation dose. Disease incidence increases proportionally with dose, and there is no dose threshold.

**Structured mottle:** A type of radiographic mottle due to variations in the structure of the intensifying screen. A factor which is spatially fixed, reproducible, not statistically variable, and the same in every image produced with a particular cassette/grid combination: grid lines visible in the image can be considered structured mottle.

**Sub-prefix:** Meaning below, under, beneath; as subnormal, sublingual, subdiaphragmatic.

**Subacute:** Between acute and chronic; having some acute symptoms.

**Subarachnoid space:** The space within the meninges between the arachnoid mater and pia mater, where cerebrospinal fluid flows.

**Subject contrast:** The part of radiographic contrast determined by the size, shape, and X-ray attenuating characteristics of the subject being examined and the energy of the X-ray beam.

**Substance:** Any drug, chemical, or biologic entity.

**Subtraction technique:** A method of removing all unnecessary anatomic structures from an image and enhancing only those of interest.

**Super-prefix:** Meaning over, above, in excess; as superimpose, supernumerary, supersaturate.

**Supercomputer:** One of the fastest and highest-capacity computers, containing hundreds to thousands of microprocessors.

**Superior:** Toward the upper part of a structure or toward the head; also called cephalic.

**Superoinferior:** Directed from above downward; craniocaudal.

**Supero-prefix:** Meaning above; situated or directed from above.

**Supervision:** Responsibility for and control of quality, radiation safety, and technical aspects of all X-ray examinations and procedures.

**Supination:** Rotation of the arm so that the palm is directed forward or anteriorly; the opposite of pronation.

**Supine:** Lying on back; opposite of prone.

**Supra- prefix:** Meaning above, higher in position; as supraclavicular, suprarenal, supraorbital.

**Target:** Material at which electrons from the cathode in an X-ray tube are aimed in order to produce X-rays.

**Target-Film Distance:** The distance from the X-ray tube target (anode) to the film measured in inches or centimeters.

**Target-Skin Distance:** The distance from the X-ray target (anode) to the skin of the patient where X-ray beam enters the body.

**Teratogenic effects:** Birth defects that are not passed on to future generations, caused by exposure to a toxin as a fetus.

**Thermoluminescent dosimeter:** A dosimeter made of certain crystalline material which is capable of both storing a fraction of absorbed ionizing radiation and releasing this energy in the form of visible photons when heated. The amount of light released can be used as a measure of radiation exposure to these crystals.

**Thermonuclear device:** A device with explosive energy that comes from fusion of small nuclei, as well as fission.

**Transmission:** Photons passing through the body.

**Umbra:** The sharp area of a radiographic image.

**Unabsorbed:** Pertaining to radiography, the term unabsorbed refers to that portion of the X-ray beam that traverses the patient and does not interact with the patient's tissues. These X-ray photons pass through the patient unaffected and expose the X-ray film, thereby contributing to the creation of the radiographic image.

**Unstable nucleus:** A nucleus that contains an uneven number of protons and neutrons and seeks to reach equilibrium between them through radioactive decay (*e.g.* the nucleus of a radioactive atom).

**Useful Beam:** Means that part of the radiation which passes through the window, aperture, cone, or other collimating device of the tube housing.

**Valence electron:** An electron in the outermost shell.

**Valgus:** Denoting a deformity in which the distal part of a limb is displaced or twisted away from the midline of the body (e.g. knock knead).

**Varus:** Denoting a deformity in which the distal part of a limb is turned inwards towards the midline of the body (e.g. bow-legged).

**Venogram:** Radiograph of veins filled with contrast medium; a phlebogram.

**Venography:** Radiologic examination of veins during injection of radiopaque solution.

**Ventrad:** Situated or directed toward abdomen or anterior aspect of body; ventrally.

**Ventral:** Toward the front or facing surface; the opposite of dorsal; also called inferior.

**Ventriculography:** Radiographic examination of brain following injection of radioparent medium into ventricles.

**Vertex:** Top or highest part of head.

**Vignetting:** A reduction in brightness at the periphery of the image.

**Viscera:** The organs within the abdominal or thoracic cavities.

**Visceral peritoneum:** A serous membrane that covers the surfaces of abdominal viscera.

**Visible light:** The radiant energy in the electromagnetic spectrum that is visible to the human eye.

**Volt (V):** The SI unit of electric potential and potential difference.

**Voltage:** A measurement of force that refers to the potential difference between two electrical charges. It determines the speed of electrons that travel from the cathode to anode, When the voltage is increased- the speed of the electrons increases, the electron strikes the target with greater force and energy, resulting in a penetrating X-ray beam with a short wavelength.

**Voxel (volume element):** Three dimensional box represented on the image matrix by the two dimensional pixel.

**Wavelength:** Determines the energy and the penetrating power of radiation. Shorter wavelengths=more penetrating power.

**Whole-body count:** The measure and analysis of the radiation being emitted from a person's entire body, detected by a counter external to the body.

**Whole-body exposure:** An exposure of the body to radiation, in which the entire body, rather than an isolated part, is irradiated by an external source.

**X-axis:** The horizontal line of a graph.

**X-radiation:** A high-energy radiation produced by the collision of a beam of electrons with a metal target in an X-ray tube.

**X-ray film:** Is composed of a clear cellulose acetate film base that is coated with an emulsion of silver halide(usually silver bromide) grains suspended in a layer of gelatin.

**X-ray generator:** A device which supplies electrical power to the X-ray tube. It does not, as the name implies, actually generate X-rays.

**X-ray imaging system:** An X-ray system designed for radiography, tomography, or fluoroscopy.

**X-ray personnel:** Individual legally allowed to use diagnostic X-rays on human beings.

**X-ray quality:** The penetrability of an X-ray beam.

**X-ray quantity:** The output intensity of an X-ray imaging system, measured in roentgens (R).

**X-ray spectrum:** The relative distribution of different energies in a photon beam. X-ray tube rating charts; Charts that guide the technologist in the use of X-ray tubes.

**X-ray:** Electromagnetic radiation caused by deflection of electrons from their original paths, or inner orbital electrons that change their orbital levels around the atomic nucleus. X-rays, like gamma rays can travel long distances through air and most other materials. Like gamma rays, X-rays require more shielding to reduce their intensity than do beta or alpha particles. X-rays and gamma rays differ primarily in their origin: X-rays originate in the electronic shell; gamma rays originate in the nucleus. Penetrating electromagnetic radiation whose wavelengths are shorter than those of visible light. X-rays are the product of the final step in the process of producing X-rays.

## Chapter - 26

# Exercise: Review Questions

The following exercises are to be answered by marking the lettered responses that best answers of the question or best completes the statement or by writing the answer. After you have completed all the exercises, turn to " Check Your Answers" at the end of the lesson. Answers are given to most of them in "Check Your Answers" except for the long types.

1. Pocket of electromagnetic energy are called............
2. Which radiology innovator is known as the father of the science of radiation protection? ..........
3. First Nobel prize in Physics received by:.............
4. In the year 1901..................received the Nobel prize in physice for the discovery of X-rays.
5. ...............is considered as father of Veterinary Radiology.
6. ................. known as the father of Interventional Radiology.
7. X-rays differ from light in that X-rays have.............
8. X-rays have a .............wevelength a........
9. X-rays that have wavelength will ......more easily than those with a...........wavelength.
10. The nucleus of an atom contains: ...................
11. Roentgen (R) is measured in .......

12. For radiographic purposes, .............are usually produced by bombarding a metallic target with fast electrons in a vacuum.
13. Where does the generation of X-rays in the X-ray tube actually occur?.......
14. What material is the most effective in stopping X-rays?..........
15. What device is used to select the kVp of an X-ray machine? .............
16. What will produce the highest contrast? ......
17. What part of the X-ray machine converts electrons to X-ray photons?.........
18. What is the primary cause of radiation damage?...............
19. Energy carried by moving electrons is measured in units of ..............
20. What is the difference between X-rays and other forms of energy found on the electromagnetic spectrum? ..............
21. What is the source of electrons used for X-ray production? .......
22. What is the best attenuator on a radiographic image?........
23. Heart of the X-ray system.........
24. Contrast is primarily a funcion of ?..........
25. .......settings determines the quality of the X-ray beam.
26. What part of the film cassette is intended to reduce patient exposure?......
27. What is used to restrict the size of the X-ray beam? .........
28. What does kV affect? ....................................
29. What does mA affect? ...................................
30. ..............determines quantity of X-ray beam production.
31. The speed at which the electrons move across an X-ray tube is regulated by .......
32. Collimator in an X-ray machine is used to decide the :a). restriction of the primary beam, b).penetration of X-rays, c).type of radiation, d.). distance of X-rays.

33. Positive terminal of the X-ray tube is called.......
34. Which part of X-ray tube is the limiting factor in the maximum energy of X-rays that can be produced: a). cathode, b).filament, c).anode, d). glass
35. Phenomenon of emission light by a phosphor crystal even after ceasation of its exposure to X-rays is known as.................
36. ..................,..................,...................,...and .......... are different types of the electromagnetic radiations while .................and ............belongs to the category of particulate radiations.
37. The ability of lead as an effective absorber of X-rays is due to its.........
38. What does density affect?................
39. When the wavelength of incident X-ray photon is same as the diameter of th target atom, the phenomenon of ..............scattering is observed.
40. The production of X-rays results in 1% X-rays and 99%: a). electrons, b). heat, c). protrons, d). ionization.
41. Both milliamperage setting and exposure time determine the ..............
42. The step up transformer is placed in the X-ray machine to convert the ...............voltage into ........voltage by a factor of ................
43. The speed at which electrons move across an X-ray tube is regulated by ........
44. Tungsten filament cathode is heated upto ...................to produce thermion and process is known as thermionic emission.
45. Increasing the milliamperage (mA) will cause .....................
46. What is the preferred exposure time for radiography of exotic animals and birds?.............
47. What method of restraint of exotic animals and birds is generally safest for the animal and handlers? A). physical, b). manual, c). chemical, d). both a and b.

48. Oil that surrounds the X-ray tube and transformers inside the tube head ...........

49. X-rays with longer wavelengths have ............penetrating power.

50. When the kilovolt peak is ......while other exposure factors remin constant, the resultant film exhibits a decreased density and appears darker?

51. X-rays with ..........are more likely to be absorbed by matter.

52. Amperage regulates the ............ of electrons produced at the cathode filament.

53. Greater penetration of xrays is obtained with ..............

54. Increasing the atomic number of the target material: a). increasing life of the tube, b). increasing the probability of electronic interactions, c). increasing the melting point, d). decreasing the cost of the machine.

55. Which cell type is the most sensitive to radiation?...................

56. The most radiosensitives tissue in the body is : a). ovaries and testis, b).muscle cells, c). fat cells, d). nerve cell.

57. What unit of radiation represents the amount of radiation energy absorbed by the tissue?............

58. What is the term used to measure the effects of different type of radiation? ......

59. Unit of radiation dose in rem is calculated by multiplying relative biological effectiveness of particular radiation to dose of radiation in :a). roentgen, b). curie, c).rads, d). Sievert.

60. What is the proper thickness of the lead lining in radiographic lead aprons and thyroid collars?.........

61. Films should be stord in a...............

62. Factors affecting the film darkness is ..............

63. ............is the unsharpness or blurred edges seen on a radiographic image.

64. A radiolucent foreign body lodged in the esophagus could be more easily seen: a). on a dorsoventral position, b).following a barium swallow, c).by making exposure during inspiration, d). by making exposure during expiration.

65. The temperature of the filament affects the: a). average energy of the X-ray produced, b). speed of the electrons produced, c). quantity of the X-rays produced.d). density of the material increased.
66. What are the applications of radiographs? ...............
67. Amount of radiation a patient receives will depends on ?
68. The lead diaphragm in the tube head is referred to as the .............
69. Where is the Placing of safelight in the darkroom..............
70. The function of grid is to: a). absorb secondary radiation, b). eliminate the need of collimator, c). reduce developing time, d). absorb primary radiation.
71. White spots in the film is caused by? ................
72. The primary purpose of sodium thiosulfate is to ..............
73. Develping time for X-ray flim is : a). 10 minute, b). 4-5 minute, c). 30-34 minute, d). 15 second
74. Secondary radiation causes in the film.......
75. Geiger muller counter is indicated to trace: a). non-radioactive element in body, b). radioisotopes in body, c). both a and b., d). useless in radioisotopes search.
76. Increasing the operating kilovoltage peak (kVp) will cause ...............
77. Which is composition of fixer: a). sodium thiosulphate, b). sodium sulphite, c). acetic acid , d). none, e). all of the above.
78. True or false. If you increase mA, you must also increase exposure time?.
79. True or false. Photoelectric effect is mostly produced when X-ray photons interact with inner shell electrons of an atom.
80. Which is compostion of developer : a). sodium sulfite, b). sodium carbonate, c). potassium bromide, d). none, e). all of the above.
81. Which technique is most suitable to brain scanning: a). Functional Magnetic resonance imaging (fMRI), b). Nuclear Scintigraphy (NS) c). single photon emission computed tomography (SPECT) d). computed tomography (CT).

82. Radiation intersity higher on the cathode side than the anode side is known as ................

83. Final washing time for X-ray film is: a). 20 -30 minute, b). 4-5 minute, c). 30-34 second, d). 20 second

84. Developing solution splashed on the film prior to processing will result in .....

85. True or false. Radiography is useful for examining post mortem material.

86. Any leaks of white light into the darkroom will cause........

87. True or false. X-rays produce phosphorence in lead acetate.

88. ............. radiation is radiation that has been deflected from its path during the impact with matter.

89. If film will be dark then it indicate condition of: a). under exposure b). over exposure, c). no exposure d). mild exposure.

90. Low kilovoltage peak settings (65-70 kVp) creates a high contrast film........

91. True or false. Large capacity X-ray units have rorating anode.

92. Where the X-unit operator stands if they cannot get 6 feet away from the patient during exposure.............

93. Portions of the X-ray unit should never be sprayed with disinfectant...............

94. Personal protective equipment to be worn during radiographic procedures:.......

95. True or false. High kVp technique chart gives greater exposure than low kVp technnique.

96. Ture or false. While taking radiograph, thicker or denser side should be positioned towards the cathode.

97. Which one of the film components is responsible for forming the image?.......

98. True or false. Hydroquinone is a good solvet for metallic silver.

99. True or false. A good technician will hold the limbs of the animal during X-ray exposure to give it comfort.

100. True or false. A rad is a measure of radiation absorption dose and is equal to absorption of 100 ergs per gram of substance.

101. What are the two major kinds of intensifying screens used radiography?
102. True or false. The exposure rate from a fluoroscope is more than that from an image intensifier.
103. True or false. X-rays can be deflected by the magnetic field.
104. True or fasle. Hard X-rays have smaller wavelength.
105. The white or light gray areas of a radiograph are referred to as .............
106. Radiographic procedure for suspected metallic foreign body in the intestine of a dog: a). barium enema, b). survey radiography, c).peumoperitoniography, d). double contrast.
107. What is the purpose of the developing solution?..............
108. Reducing agents in the developer change silver bromide crystals to black metallic silver and also act as electron donors to the latent image site. In this latter function, their action results in a: a). Negative charge in the exposed area. b). Positive charge in the exposed area, c). Softening of the gelatin base. d). Release of secondary radiation.
109. What is the purpose of the restrainer in the developing solution?
110. An appropriate safelight filter should be positioned at least ......feet away from the counter top and contain a light bulb no bigger than .........watts.
111. What is the main purpose of the fixing solution?.......
112. True or false. Phosphate calculi are radiopaque while urate and cystine calculi are radioluncent.
113. True or false. Reticular abscess gives blackish density in the plain radiography.
114. True or false. The main ingredient in the developer is an oxidizing agent.
115. True or false. The wave length of the diagnostic X-ray is about $10^{-8}$.
116. True or false. Use of intensifying screens causes some lose of details and definition in the radiographs.
117. Aluminum filters are placed in the path of the beam to ...........

118. An overdeveloped radiograph will produce an image that is ........than a normal radiograph.
119. Contrast radiography of the renal architecture is known as .......
120. A blurred or fuzzy image will be produced by .......
121. What is ALARA? ......................................
122. True or false. Ovaries are less sensitive than testes to the radiation.
123. True or false. Intravenous pyelography can be used for diagonise of renal parenchymatous tumours.
124. True or false. Pregnancy in the canine can be assessed radiographically at four weeks of gestation.
125. 10 mA for .6 = 15 mA for ...........s?
126. Irradiation of hands by careless use of diagnostic radiographic equipment will increase the chance of development of .................of skin.
127. Name the contrast technique and the contrast agents for teat canal of a cow: .......
128. Fixing a radiograph for several hours may produce a radiograph that appears ..........than normal.
129. The capability of the receptor to reproduce distinct outlines of an object is called? ...
130. Identify the term that describes how dark and light areas are differentiated on an image............
131. True or false. Gastrography should not be performed in dogs suffering from diabetes mellitus.
132. The overall blackness or darkness of an image .......
133. One milliampere is equal to ............of an ampere.
134. Therapeutic use of radioisotopes within the interstitium or on the surface of a tumour is known as ..............
135. The portion of processed radiograph that appears dark or black is? .........
136. The portion of a processed radiograpgh that appears light or white is? .........

137. Define the following: a). absorbed dose, b). radiation dose, c). quality factor.

138. What are 10 characteristics of an X-ray?

139. Material used most commonly for ultrasound transducer is: a). lead zirconate titanate, b). zinc cobalt titanate, c). lead ferro zirconate, d). lead titanium dioxide.

140. What are 3 exposure factor?

141. Write down the manual film processing steps..............

142. Lethal dose: LD- 50/30, means....................

143. 1 Sv( Sievert ) is equal to ... .... rem.

144. Which of the following renal stone does not cast shadow in plain X-ray:a). phosphate, b). uric acid, c). oxalate, d). none.

145. As the density of a tissue increases, the amount of scatter produced: a). doubles, b). decreases,c). remain contast, d). increases.

146. When compared with the bone, attenuation of kidney tissue is: a). lower, b). higher, c). identical, d). none of the above.

147. True or false. The siver halide grains react to form th latent image.

148. During radiotherapy the radiation effect can more reliabily be known by estimating the number of : a). thrombocytes, b). lymphocytes, c). polymorpho nuclear lymphocytes, d). erythrocytes

149. What will be the new mAs if the FFD is changed from75 cm to 90 cm and the original mAs was 20.

150. If the mA is 70 and the time is 0.4 seconds, what mAs is being used?

151. If an mA of 30 and a time of 0.4 seconds are used to radiographed a dog metatarsus with kV of 50, what exposure factors are used?

152. The intensify screen is used to: a). reduce patient dose, b). increase patient dose c). replace X-rays film d). convert electricity to light.

153. Which one of the following elements is used for MRI studies: a). Hydrogen, b). Carbon, c). Oxygen, d). Nitrogen.

154. True or false. Developer decreases the sensitized silver halides to bromine.

155. True or false: water is used as the solvent in processing because it is cheap.

156. First step of film processing is: a). developing, b). fixing, c).drying d). washing.

157. The tissues most susceptible to radiation damage are: a). red blood cells, b). muscle c). bone. d). skin.

158. Lead is generally used as a filter material in: a).cobalt beam physiotherapy unit, b).granz ray therapy unit, c).deep physiotherapy unit, d).contact physiotherapy unit.

159. The technique that uses X-rays to produce an image is: a). magnetic resonance imaging, b).computerised tomography, c). digital imaging d).ultrasound.

160. The definition of kilovoltage (kV) is the:a). current of X-rays, b).quality of X-rays, c).time of X-rays. d).penetrating power of X-rays.

161. Which one of the following is used for personnel monitoring of radiation: a). pocket dosimeter, b).geiger muller counter, c).thermoluminescence dosimeter, d).air ionization chamber.

162. True or false. MRI is not suitable for the diagnosis of intracranial mass lesions.

163. The imaging technique that uses X-rays to produe an image is: a). ultrasound, b).digital imaging, c).MRI, d).CT

164. A Potter Bucky diaphragm is an example of a: a). moving grid, b).focussed grid, c).stationary grid, d).pseudofocused grid.

165. The grid factor relates to the amount by which the: a). mAs must be increased, b). mAs must be decreased, c).kV must be increased, d), kV must be decreased.

166. True or false. Doppler ultrasonography is only applicable for measuring blood flow in great vessels.

167. The type of waves that ultrasound uses to form an image are:a).light, b).sound, c).visible, d).ultraviolet.

168. True or false. Beta rays are more penetrative than alfa rays.

169. An intravenous urogram is a contrast study of the: a).urinary system, b).reproductive sytem, c). neurological system, d). circulatory system.

170. Write radiological diagnosis of intussusceptions in a dog.

171. The dose equivalent in rems is equal to the absorbed dose in .......multiplied by the quality factor.

172. Who has invented grid?.............

173. Radiation intensity higher on the cathode side than the anode side is known as ..............

174. Write in short the advantages of computer applications in veterinary surgical research.

175. Biological effect of X-ray used fo the treatment of cancer is based on its affinity towards : a). fast multiplying cells, b). generating cells, c). degeranative cells, d). none.

176. In radiographic exposure parameters, one of the following is considered contant: a). part film distance, b). time, c). kVp, d). mA.

177. True or false: ultrasonic waves increase the membrane permeability which increase fluid absorption.

178. Radiographic appreacnce of foreing body obstruction of pylorus in dog is: a). Distension of stomach, b). distended intestinal loop, c). sacculations of intestinal loop d). none of the above.

179. Collimator in an X-ray machine is used to decide the : a). type of radiation, b). distance of X-rays. c). field of radiation. d). direction of X-rays.

180. Father of veterinary radiology is :a). stator, b). Eberlein, c). roentegon, d). kirschner.

181. Nuclear scientigraphy uses the emission of which part of the electromagnetic spectrum to form an image: a). gamma rays, b). infrared, c). beta rays, d). alpha rays.

182. Malignant tumors are more .........to radiotherapy because of increased ............

183. Difference in intensity across the X-ray beam is called:a). knee effect, b). heel effect, c). Keel effect, d). kneil effect.

184. What method of diagnostic imaging evaluates the cardiac wall and valvular movement in real time..................

185. Ultrasonic waves can be used for examing the properties of small quantities of matter because of their..........

186. Which of the following can be detected with the help of ultrasonography: a). hepatic mass, b).peristalsis, c). non-pregnant reproductive tract, d). both a and b.

187. What is the most suitable and common way to diagnostic hyperthyroidism in cat.................

188. Rate the echogenicity of the following with the first being most echogenic and the last being the least echogenic: Spleen, liver, renal cortex.

189. True or false. Doppler sound effect occurs when the structures distance between the sound recorder and the source of sound changes with time.

190. Which of the following would cause acoustic shadowing: a). urine, b). bone, c). air in the stomach, d). free blood in the abdomen.

191. False or True. Anechoic tissue reflects more echoes than hyperechoic tissue.

192. X-rays have their greatest harmful effect upon: a). skin, b). lung, c). gonadal part, d). bone.

193. True or false. In CAT scan time can be reduced by using several pencil sized beams and an array of detectors.

194. X-ray film must be characteristically different from photographic film because: a). X-ray specialist are not trained in photography, b). X-ray exposure is different from light exposure, c). It is used under different temperature conditions, d). It is susceptible to high humidity.

195. In X-ray film, the film base is usually composed of polyester or: a). Silver bromide, b). Emulsion, c). Cellulose acetate, d). Gelatin.

196. In ultrasonography movement of organs can be studied in : a). real time scan image, b). A-mode scan image, c). B-mode scan image, d). none of the above.

197. What suspension material is used to hold the silver bromide crystals? a). Cotton cellulose. b). Cellulose acetate. c). Silver iodine. d). Gelatin.

198. When X-rays are taken using intensifying screens, account(s) for most of the exposure: a). X-rays. b). Gamma rays. c). Beta rays. d). Fluorescent light.

199. Geiger-muller counter is mainly used as a radiation: a). detector, b). monitor, c). personel monitor, d). detector as well as monitor.

200. The emulsion X-ray film is coated with a thin, transparent material to: a). Allow visual inspection of the latent image, b). Allow the passage of light, c). Protect it during handling and storage, d). Maintain the purity of the emulsion.

201. Because of the chemicals released by the developing process, which of the following ingredients included in a fresh developer solution is not used in the replenisher? a). Elon™, b). Potassium bromide, c). Sodium sulfite, d).Hydroquinone.

202. Computerized tomographic value for water is: a). 20-25, b). -100, c). 0, d). 100

203. In the developer solution, sodium sulfite works well as preservative because it: a). increases the activity of the reducing agents, b). reduces oxidation of the reducing agents, c). allows the reducers to work at a higher temperature, d). none.

204. Double bubble is a characteristic radiographic appearance in ..........

205. Who invented the CAT and when?

206. When used with conventional X-ray film, safelight filters should be: a). red, b). green, c). yellow, d). blue.

207. What is a pixel and voxel?

208. Write short notes on: a). digital imaging, b). MRI, c). CAT, d). teletherapy, e). transducer.

209. Match the following ;

| | |
|---|---|
| 1. X-ray: | dark |
| 2. X-ray tube: | created when primary interact with matter |
| 3. Underdeveloped film: | light |
| 4. Tubehead: | created when X-ray that comes from tube |
| 5. Short scale contrast: | scattered radiation |
| 6. Secondary radiation: | vacuum tube in which X-rays are produced |
| 7. Scatter radiation : | invisible, odorless electromagnetic radiation |
| 8. Primary radiation : | where the X-ray tube and transformers are located |
| 9. overdeveloped film: | image sharpness |
| 10. mA: | shows only two densities, black and white |
| 11. Long scale contrast: | created when X-ray deflect from path by matter |
| 12. kVp: | number of electrons produced |
| 13. intensifying screen: | many shades of gray (higher kVp, low contrast) |
| 14. grid: | number of electrons |
| 15. Exposure time: | speed of electrons |
| 16. Control panel: | Positive electrode |
| 17. collimator : | X-ray beam restrictor |
| 18. Central Beam: | the primary ray emitting from the X-ray machine: |
| 19. Collimator: | Negative electrode |
| 20. Cathode: | a device used to eliminate peripheral radiation |
| 21. Anode: | controls the operating system of X-ray machine |

210. Match the following:

| | | |
|---|---|---|
| a. | Sodium hydroxide: | restrainer |
| b. | Protective layer: | coating over emulsion |
| c. | Potassium bromide: | adhesive material |
| d. | Hydroquinone: | plastic |
| e. | Film emulsion: | accelerator |
| f. | Film base: | developing agent |
| g. | Adhesive layer: | coating on film base |

211. Match the following:

| | | |
|---|---|---|
| i. | Decrease focal spot size: | greater loss of image sharpness. |
| ii. | Increase crystal size : | sharper image appears |
| iii. | Longer wavelengths : | more power. |
| iv. | Shorter wavelengths : | less power |
| v. | smaller the focal spot area: | sharpness decrease. |
| vi. | larger the focal spot area: | sharpness increase |

212. Match the following:

| | | |
|---|---|---|
| A. | protons: | dense core of the atom |
| B. | neutron: | fundamental unit of matter |
| C. | nucleus: | positive charged particles |
| D. | electrons: | particles with no charge |
| E. | atom: | 3 kev |
| F. | k shell electrons: | 12 kev |
| G. | L shell electrons: | 70 kev |
| H. | M shell electrons: | negatively charged particles |

213. Match the following:

| | | |
|---|---|---|
| i. | Developing time: | 15 minutes |
| ii. | Rinsing time: | 30 minutes |
| iii. | Fixing time: | 5 mintues |
| iv. | Drying time: | 30 seconds |

214. Match the following:

| | |
|---|---|
| a. Barium: | used for arthrography |
| b. Iodine in water: | used in magnetic resonance imaging. |
| c. Magnevist: | used to make parts of the gastrointestinal tract opaque. |
| d. Sterile saline (salt water): | double contrast |
| e. Contrast radiography of esophagus : | myelography |
| f. Contrast radiography of spinal cord architecture: | bronchography |
| g. Contrast radiography of broanchus: | oesophagography |
| h. Cystography: | used during hysterosonography. |

## Chapter - 27

# Check Your Answers

1. Photons.
2. Wilhelm Conrad Roentgen
3. Wilhelm Conrad Roentgen, Bavarian physicist discovered the X-ray on November 8, 1895.
4. Wilhelm Conrad Roentgen
5. Richard Eberlein
6. Charles Dotter
7. more energy
8. short, high
9. penetrate
10. protons and neutrons
11. Air
12. X-rays
13. Tungsten (target)
14. Lead
15. autotransformer
16. Low kVp
17. The anode
18. Ionization

19. Electrons volts
20. Wavelength and frequency are different.
21. Tungsten filament
22. Lead
23. X-ray tube
24. kVp
25. kVp
26. intensifying screen.
27. Collimation
28. penetrating power, speed of electrons from cathode to anode, and radiographic contrast.
29. amount of radiation and temperature of the cathode
30. mAs
31. kilovoltage
32. a). restriction of the primary beam
33. Anode (target)
34. c).anode
35. phosphorescence
36. visible light,ultravioliet, gamma rays, X-rays radio waves and heat waves, alpha and beta
37. high atomic number.
38. darkness of a film
39. coherent
40. b). heat
41. number of X rays produced
42. predicted , high, 1000.
43. kilovoltage
44. 2200 -2800 $^{0}$
45. an increase in density; the film appears darker
46. 1/40 or less
47. c).chemical

48. insulating oil
49. less
50. increased
51. longer wavelengths
52. quantity
53. increased kVp
54. b). increasing the probability of electronic interactions
55. immature cells
56. a). ovaries and testis
57. Gray
58. Sievert
59. c).rads
60. 0.25 mm equivalent
61. cool and dry location
62. exposure time, mA, target-film distance, size of patient, and processing conditions.
63. Penumbra
64. b).following a barium swallow
65. c). quantity of the X-rays produced
66. to detect diseases that may be left undetected with an clinical exam.
67. exposure time and mA
68. collimator
69. a minimum of 4 feet from the film and working area
70. a). absorb secondary radiation
71. fixer spill
72. remove the silver bromide crystals that have not been developed and enhance contrast
73. b). 4-5 minute
74. film fog
75. b). radioisotopes in body

76. an increase in density; the film appears darke
77. e. all of the above
78. False. An increase in mA needs a decrease in exposure time.
79. True
80. e). all of the above.
81. a). Functional Magnetic resonance imaging (fMRI)
82. heel effect
83. a). 20 -30 minute
84. dark spots
85. True
86. film fog
87. false
88. Scatter
89. b). over exposure
90. many black and white areas, few shades of gray
91. true
92. behind an appropriate barrier or outside.
93. electrical areas (ex. control panel, switches)
94. gloves
95. false
96. ture
97. silver halide crystals
98. false
99. false
100. true
101. rare earth and calcium tungstate
102. true
103. false
104. true
105. radiopaque

106. b). survey radiography
107. swell and soften the emulsion of the film; develop silver halide crystals containing latent image
108. a). Negative charge in the exposed area
109. prevents the developing agents from acting on the silver halide crystals that do not contain a latent image
110. 4; 15
111. Remove all underdeveloped sliver halide crystals from the emulsion; shrink and harden emulsion to prevent from scratching
112. True
113. True
114. False
115. True
116. True
117. reduce intensity.
118. Darker
119. intravenous pyelography
120. movement
121. As low as reasonably achievable
122. False
123. False
124. True.
125. 0.4
126. squamous cell carcinoma
127. thallography, air
128. lighter
129. sharpness
130. contrast
131. true
132. density

133. 1/1000
134. brachytherapy
135. radiolucent
136. radiopaque
137. a. This is a measure of the amount of energy absorbed from the radiation beam per unit mass of tissue. b. Units of energy absorption per unit mass (joules/kg) called the gray (rad).c. the biological effects of different radiations, provides a common unit for comparison of different type of radiations for X-rays quality factor is 1 and for Alpha particles quality factor is 20
138. From the book.
139. a). lead zirconate titanate,
140. kVp (kilovolt peak), mA, Exposure time (second).
141. 1.development- reduces exposed, energized crystals chemically into black metallic silver. It softens film emulsion during process, 2. rinse- removes the developer from the film and stops the development process, 3. fixing- remove the unexposed, unenergized silver halide crystals from the film emulsion. It hardens the film emulsion, 4. washing- water bath to wash film. removes excess chemicals, 5. drying-must completely dry
142. LD- 50/30, means kill 50% of the population in 30 days
143. 100
144. b).uric acid,
145. d). increases.
146. a). lower
147. true
148. a). thrombocytes
149. 28.8.
150. 28.
151. 12 mAs and 50 kV.
152. a). reduce patient dose
153. a). Hydrogen

154. False
155. True
156. a). developing
157. a). red blood cells
158. a).cobalt beam physiotherapy unit,
159. b).computerised tomography
160. d).penetrating power of X-rays.
161. a). pocket dosimeter,
162. False
163. d).CT
164. a). moving grid
165. a). mAs must be increased
166. false
167. b).sound
168. false
169. a).urinary system
170. see text.
171. Rads
172. Gustav Bucky
173. heel effect.
174. **Ans:** a). Easy collection of data both from the eqiupement and monitoring systems of the patient. b). Observation can be ananylised or manipulated an any conceivable type of biomedical research projects. c). Reduce the time and experimental animals required and analysis of the different variable. d). Multidimentional statistical testing. e). Modeling, stimulation and prediction on various aspect of bioengineering. f). Three dimensional mapping of normal anatomy, modeling of cells and tissue morphology. g). Easy access of bibliographical and research information helps in proper planning and formulation of research program.
175. a). fast multiplying cells
176. a). part film distance

177. true
178. a). Distension of stomach,
179. c. field of radiation
180. b. Eberlein
181. : a).gamma rays
182. susceptible , metabolism
183. b). heel effect,
184. M-mode ultranosography.
185. Shortwave length
186. d). both a and b.
187. nuclear scientigrphy
188. spleen (most) ,liver, renal cortex (least).
189. True
190. b).bone,
191. false
192. c). gonadal part
193. True.
194. b). X-ray exposure is different from light exposure.
195. c). Cellulose acetate.
196. a). real time scan
197. d). Gelatin.
198. d). Fluorescent light.
199. a). detector
200. c). Protect it during handling and storage,
201. b). Potassium bromide
202. c).0
203. b). reduces oxidation of the reducing agents.
204. GDV
205. G. N. Hounsfield in 1972.
206. a). red

207. Pixel: Picture elements (each square in the image matrix), Voxel: tiny alongated block of tissue

208. From the text.

209. Match the following ;

| | |
|---|---|
| 1. X-ray: | invisible, odorless electromagnetic radiation |
| 2. X-ray tube: | vacuum tube in which X-rays are produced |
| 3. Underdeveloped film: | light |
| 4. Tubehead: | where the X-ray tube and transformers are located |
| 5. Short scale contrast: | shows only two densities, black and white |
| 6. Secondary radiation: | created when primary interact with matter |
| 7. Scatter radiation : | created when X-ray deflect from path by matter |
| 8. Primary radiation : | created when X-ray that comes from tube |
| 9. overdeveloped film: | dark |
| 10. mA: | number of electrons |
| 11. Long scale contrast: | many shades of gray (higher kVp, low contrast) |
| 12. kVp: | speed of electrons |
| 13. intensifying screen: | image sharpness |
| 14. grid: | scattered radiation |
| 15. Exposure time: | number of electrons produced |
| 16. Control panel: | device that controls the operating system of X-ray machine |
| 17. collimator : | X-ray beam restrictor |
| 18. Central Beam: | the primary ray emitting from the X-ray machine: |

19. Collimator: a device used to eliminate peripheral radiation
20. Cathode: Negative electrode
21. Anode: Positive electrode

210. Match the following:

a. Sodium hydroxide: accelerator
b. Protective layer : coating over emulsion
c. Potassium bromide: restrainer
d. Hydroquinone: developing agent
e. Film emulsion: coating on film base
f. Film base: plastic
g. Adhesive layer: adhesive material

211. Match the following:

i. Decrease focal spot size: sharpness increase
ii. Increase crystal size : sharpness decrease
iii. Longer wavelengths : less power.
iv. Shorter wavelengths : more power.
v. smaller the focal spot area: sharper image appears.
vi. larger the focal spot area: greater loss of image sharpness.

212. Match the following:

A. protons: positive charged particles
B. neutron: particles with no charge
C. nucleus: dense core of the atom
D. electrons: negatively charged particles
E. atom: fundamental unit of matter
F. k shell electrons: 70 kev
G. L shell electrons: 12 kev
H. M shell electrons: 3 kev

213. Match the following:

| | | |
|---|---|---|
| i. | Developing time: | 5 mintues |
| ii. | Rinsing time: | 30 seconds |
| iii. | Fixing time: | 15 minutes |
| iv. | Drying time: | 30 minutes |

214. Match the following:

| | | |
|---|---|---|
| a. | Barium: | used to make parts of the gastrointestinal tract opaque. |
| b. | Iodine in water: | used for arthrography. |
| c. | Magnevist: | used in magnetic resonance imaging. |
| d. | Sterile saline (salt water): | used during hysterosonography. |
| e. | Contrast radiography of esophagus : | oesophagography |
| f. | Contrast radiography of spinal cord architecture: | myelography |
| g. | Contrast radiography of broanchus: | bronchography |
| h. | Cystography: | double contrast |

# Chapter - 28

# References/Selected Readings

Ansari, M.M. 2011. Advances and application of diagnostic ultrasonography in Veterinary practice-a review. *Livestock Line.* 5 (3): 11-14.

Ansari, M.M. 2013. Myelography in Veterinary Practice. Handbook on short course on diagnostic imaging, SKUAST-K, Srinagar, pp 28-34.

Ansari, M.M. 2013. Contrast enhanced unltrasonography. Handbook on short course on diagnostic imaging, SKUAST, Srinagar, pp 64-73.

Becher, H and Burns, P.N. 2000. *Handbook of Contrast Echocardiography.* Berlin: Springer Verlag.

Bojrab, M. J., Ellison,G.W. and Barclay, S. 1998. Current techniques in small animal surgery. 4th edition, William and Wilkins, A Waverly Company, London.

Bowden, C. and Masters, J. 2002. Quick reference guide to veterinary radiography kits. Butterworth Heinemann Publisher, New York.

Bushberg, J.T., Seibert, J.A., Leidholdt, E.M and Boone.J.M .2002. The essential physics of medical imaging, Second edition,Lippincott Williams and Wilkins, pp 1-15.

Connor, J.J.O.2005. Veterinary Surgery. 4th edition, CBS Publishers and Distributors, Delhi-110032.

Denny, P. P. and Heaton, B. 1999. Physics for Diagnostic Radiology. USA: CRC Press.

DileepKumar, K.M. and Ansari, M.M. 2011. Computed tomography (CT) in Veterinary practice –a review. *Livestock Line.* 5 (7): 9-14.

Douglas, S.W., Herrtage, M.E. and Williamson, H.D. 1987. Priniciple of veterinary radiography, 4th edn, Bariiere Tindal, London.

Easton, S. 2006. Veterinay radiography a workbook for students. Elsvier Butterworth Heinemann Publisher, New York.

Frank, E.R. 2002. Veterinary Surgery. 7th edition, CBS Publishers and Distributors, Delhi-110032.

Goldberg, B.B. 1997.Ultrasound contrast agents. London: Martin Dunitz,

Gugjoo, M.B., M., Zama, M.S.S., Saxena, A.C., Pawde, A.M. Ansari, M.M. and Bhat, S.A. 2013. Vertebral scale system to measure heart size on thoracic radiographs of Labrador retriever dogs. *Indian Veterinary Journal.* 90(2): 71-73.

Han, M.C. and Hurd, C.D. 2005. Practical diagnostic imaging for the veterinary technician. 3rd edition, Elsevier Mosby, Missouri-63146.

Hathcock. J. T and Stickle. R. L. 1993. Principles and concepts of computed tomography. The Veterinary clinics of North America. *Small Animal Practice* 23 (2) : 399-415.

http://www.hillagric.ac.in./edu/covas/vsr/radiology.

Jerrold, T., Bushberg, J., Anthony S., Edwin M. L. and John, M. B 2002. The essential physics of medical imaging. Lippincott Williams & Wilkins.

Karlsson, E. B. 2000. The Nobel Prizes in Physics 1901–2000. Stockholm: The Nobel Foundation. Retrieved 24 November 2011.

Leighton, T.G. 1994. The Acoustic Bubble. New York: Academic Press;

Lindner, J.R. 2004. Microbubbles in medical imaging: current applications and future directions. *Nat Rev Drug Discov.* 3: 527-32.

Morgan, J.P., Silverman, S. 1993. Technique of Veterinary Radiography, 5th edn., Davis, California.

Novelline, R. 1997. Squire's Fundamentals of Radiology. 5th edn., Harvard University Press.

Nyland, T.G. and Marroon, J.S. 2002. Veterinary Diagnostic Ultrasound. 2nd ed. Philadelphia, Lea and Fabiger.

Ohlerth, S. and Scharf, G. 2007. Computed tomography in small animals—basic principles and state of the art applications. *Vet. J.* 173(2):254-271.

Ryan, G.D. 1981. Radiographic technique of small animals, Philadelphia, Lea and Fabiger.

Shubik P. 1982. Vascularization of tumors: a review. *J Cancer Res Clin Oncol*; 103:211–216.

Singh, A.P. and Singh, J. 1984. Veterinary Radiology-basic principle and radiographic poistioning, CBS Publishers and Distributors, Delhi.

Singh, G.R. and Hoque, M. 2004. Manual on veterinary radiology, Division of surgery, IVRI, Izatnagar-243122, UP.

Stockley, S . 1986. A Manual of radiographic equipment. London, Churchill Livingstone.

Swaim, S.F. and Handerson, R.A.Jr.1997. Small animal wound management. 2nd edition, William and Wilkins, A Waverly company, London.

Thrall, D.E. 1998. Textbook of veterinary diagnostic radiology, 3rd edn, W.B. Saunders, Co. Philadelphia.

Ticer, J.W. 1984. Radiographic technique in veterinary practice, 2nd edn, Philadelphia, Saunders.

Toll, R.L. 1992. Ultrasound for the practitioner. Wallingford, Conn, Corometrics, Medical Systems.

Venugopalan, A. 2000. Essentials of veterinary surgery, 8th edition; Oxford and IBH, New Delhi. 110002.

Whaites, E. and Roderick, C. 2002. Essentials of Dental Radiography and Radiology. Elsevier Health Sciences.

## Chapter - 29

# Appendix

**X-ray Report Format/Requisition Slip**

Name of the Department

Name and address of Institution

---

Case receipt no........................ Date.....................

Film no........................ Envelope no.................

**Case report**

Unit: Medicine/Surgery/obstetric & Gyneacology OP/IP

Case no..........................

Name and address of the owner .............................................................................................Mobile no.........................................

Species................breed.................sex..................age...........

Part/area to be radiographed:

Skull: cranium, sinus, temporo-mandibular joint, mandible

Spine: cervical spine, thoraro-lumber (TL)spine, pelvis, sacrum

Forelimbs: (left/ right): scapula, shoulder joint, humerus, elbow joint, radius ulna, carpus and metacarpus, digits.

Hind limbs: (left/right): pelvis, hip joint, femur, stifle joint, tibia fibula, tarsus and metatarsus, digists.

Neck: Thorax: Abdomen: Bladder: Urethra:

Position/view(s) ..........................................................................

Special technique required if any.................................................

History (signs/symptoms, duration of ailment, treatment given if

any)......................................................................................................
..................................................................................................................
Tentative diagnosis ......................................................................................

**(Surgeon /Clinician)**

---

X-ray report:

Case no.: Date: X-ray ref.no.: Part X-rayed:

Radiographic quality: Good/adequate/poor/requires re-exposure

Radiographic interpretation........................

Result/Diagnosis...................................................

**(Radiologist)**

***Note:***

- *The report is not valid for medico-legal case.*
- *The clinicians are advised to correlated the findings clinically too.*